Acupuncture Points
IMAGES & FUNCTIONS

Acupuncture Points

IMAGES & FUNCTIONS

by Arnie Lade

To my family

©1989 by Eastland Press, Inc.
P.O. Box 99749, Seattle, WA 98139 USA
www.eastlandpress.com

All rights reserved. No part of this book may be reproduced or transmitted in any form or by any means, electronic or mechanical, including photocopying, recording, or by any information storage and retrieval system, without the prior written permission of the publisher, except where permitted by law

Library of Congress Catalog Card Number: 88-82703
International Standard Book Number: 0-939616-50-5

First softcover edition 2005

2   4   6   8   10   9   7   5   3

Printed in the United States of America
by Cushing-Malloy, Inc.
Ann Arbor, Michigan

Brush calligraphy by Yuki Karsten
Book design by Catherine L. Nelson & Gary Niemeier

Table of Contents

Foreword vii
Acknowledgments ix
Introduction xi

♦

Chapter 1: Point Function Terminology 1
Chapter 2: Point Classification 7
Chapter 3: Point Images and Functions................... 27
Chapter 4: Point Function Repertory 311

♦

Appendix I: Character Dictionary 329
Appendix II: Point Index 355
Bibliography 359

Foreword

During the last decade, our knowledge in the West about acupuncture and other aspects of traditional Oriental medicine has grown very quickly. Basic and intermediate texts have been published, specialized fields have developed, and the acceptance of acupuncture has spread through much of Europe, Australia, and the United States.

During this process a creative tension has developed between the acupuncture profession in the West and those of the major east Asian countries where acupuncture has been practiced for thousands of years. Each of the Asian countries tries to claim a preeminent place for its own traditions and styles in defining the theory and practice of acupuncture. To some extent, each of these claims has been accepted by various groups in the West. On the other hand, Westerners as a group consider ourselves to be very quick learners, and like to think of ourselves as being in the vanguard of progress. This has led some of us to maintain that acupuncture will only truly come into full flower here in the West.

A correct appreciation of where acupuncture has come from, its present state, and its future direction requires that we come to terms with all these paradoxical currents. Acupuncture originated in ancient China, but as it spread and developed throughout east Asia over a period of fifteen hundred to two thousand years, each country made its own distinctive contributions. These adaptations and developments reflect the unique aspects of each country's culture and people. In a similar fashion, we in the West have begun to utilize and adapt what we feel is valuable from all of these traditions, and to make our own contributions.

Part of the gulf that still separates East from West and past from present in the world of acupuncture can be attributed to language. Even in a "hands-on" healing art, a practitioner's depth of understanding is in some important ways determined by how well she or he comprehends the terminology used in that art. What cannot be conceived cannot be understood. When information and knowledge are transferred from one group to another, each with its own culture and gaze, something is always lost. This is a particularly difficult problem in traditional oriental medicine where the differences between the world view and culture of the ancient Chinese and the modern West are so great as to appear insurmountable.

Translation of the acupuncture point names is a good illustration of this problem. Most Western practitioners prefer to use a numbering system to refer to the points, and with good reason. It is systematic, logical, easy to learn, and helps us to focus on the channels. The drawback to using this type of system is that we lose the information that the point names convey, including the images they suggest. The detailed descriptions of these images in *Acupuncture Points: Images & Functions* not only tell us about the functions of the points, they are also a door through which we can glimpse the sensibility of the ancient acupuncturists. This information is complemented by the cataloging of the traditional functions of the points, and the indications for their use.

Many previous translations of the point names into English suffer from a certain superficiality, or from a lack of clinical perspective. That is not the case here. This book is the result of exensive research into Chinese, Japanese, and Western sources, the collaboration between the author and respected practitioners and translators in China, and the clinical experience of the author himself. Although not intended to be the last word on the subject, it is certain to deepen our understanding of the vision of ancient Chinese practitioners, and to enhance our ability to apply that vision in the care of the sick.

Dan Bensky
January 1989
Seattle

Acknowledgments

This work would have been incomplete without the assistance of two friends and colleagues: Su Zhi-hong, author and eminent medical translator with the Beijing International Acupuncture Training Center, and Yang Jian-feng, Director of the Acupuncture and Moxibustion Department at the Chengdu College of Traditional Chinese Medicine. Their review, support and criticism made this task possible. In particular, I thank Madame Su for her help with point name translation and Dr. Yang for his assistance in reviewing point functions and associated symptoms.

I also extend thanks to Dr. Wee-chong Tan and Dr. Ron Puhky of the Canadian College for Chinese Studies for providing a fellowship and for giving me encouragement and support in completing this manuscript. I am very grateful to Dr. Tao Jing-song of the Shanghai College of Traditional Chinese Medicine for his kindness in clarifying the finer details of function terminology. Special thanks to Nissi Wang for her expert editorial advice and to Dan Bensky for his enthusiasm and support for this project.

Introduction

The purpose of this book is to provide the student and practitioner of traditional Chinese medicine with an explanation of the images and functions of the major acupuncture points. Images are the mental pictures formed from the meanings of the characters which comprise the name of a point; functions are the energetic actions of the point itself. The information presented, especially the interpretation of the point images, is not meant to be definitive, but to provide the reader with a foundation for internalizing the images and corresponding functions of the points.

The Chinese language with its subtle use of imagery and inference makes the translation of the point names especially difficult. Like poetry, the meaning of the point names, rooted in ancient tradition, is open to interpretation. And although there is a consensus about the meaning of some names, there is disagreement about others. In keeping with the practical focus of this work, various interpretations (including my own) have been included whenever relevant or useful.

In recent years, the functions or actions of the acupuncture points have been the focus of increased attention in the literature. Although some view this as a new development, in fact, such descriptions date back to the formative era of Chinese medicine. For example, there are passages in the *Classic of Difficulties (Nan jing)* which allude to point function: "Spring points master body heat" *(ying zhu shen re)* and "Sea points master rebellious Qi as well as diarrhea" *(he zhu ni qi er chang)*. Many of the later medical classics also mention the functions of the points, but never in any systematic fashion. That task has been left to the modern era. During the last thirty years, much progress has been made in delineating the various functions of the points and their relationship to specific symptoms and patterns. This has provided the practitioner with a valuable tool in understanding the full range of point dynamics.

Approximately 250 of the most widely-used points have been selected for this book. Chapter 1, which discusses point function terminology, and chapter 2, which explains point classification, provide the background for the images and functions of the points discussed in chapter 3. Forming the main body of the book, this chapter includes the classification, location, images, functions, associated indications, and contraindications of each of the points. In most cases, examples of symptoms, patterns, or disorders have been provided to illustrate how a function or group of functions may be practically applied or further differentiated in the clinic. Chapter 4, organized in table form, provides a quick reference to the full repertory of functions and their associated primary (commonly used) and secondary points. Appendix I, a dictionary of the individual Chinese characters, lists those points whose names share the same characters, distinguishes characters with several meanings, and highlights translations used in the text. Appendix II is an index of the points which is arranged according to channel (Lung), number (L-5), pinyin *(chǐ zé)*, and translation (Cubit Marsh).

Throughout the text, two symbols are used to signify that either moxibustion$^{(\triangle)}$ or bloodletting$^{(\bigcirc)}$ rather than needling is indicated for a particular function.

May this work serve the student and practitioner well in his or her effort to help others.

CHAPTER 1

Point Function Terminology

This chapter introduces the words and phrases used to describe the functions or actions of the points. In translating the functions, English words and phrases that best retain the meaning, form, and usage of the original Chinese have been chosen. Chinese compound phrases such as "dispels Wind and clears Heat" (*qu feng qing re*) have been simplified to "dispels Wind-Heat" in order to isolate a particular point function with a specific syndrome. In some cases, a phrase such as *shu gan*, which literally means "spreads the Liver," has been amplified to "spreads Liver Qi" to capture the full meaning. Chinese characters such as *tong* translate into different words depending on context: "facilitates" Qi flow, "clears" the nose, and "unblocks" the Blood vessels. Conversely, a single English word like "benefit" may encompass several Chinese characters: *li she* (benefits the tongue), *jian nao* (benefits the Brain), and *cong er* (benefits the ears). In other instances, where several functions may relate to a single pattern (such as Dampness), specific verbs are used to describe the different functions: transforms Dampness (*hua shi*), resolves Dampness (*li shi*), and dries Dampness (*zao shi*). Terms chosen to describe a function may also identify the location of a pattern: "dispels Cold" refers to exterior Cold; "warms Cold" refers to interior Cold.

Alleviates (*jiě*) 解
relieves pain (*jie tong*).

Benefits
(*li*) 利
improves vitality, makes smooth, and restores normal functioning of the diaphragm (*li ge*), tongue (*li she*), joints (*hua li guan jie*), shoulder (*li jian*), and hip (*li bi shu*).

(*jiàn*) 健
strengthens and invigorates the transforming and transporting function of the Spleen (*jian pi*); increases and restores strength and vitality to the back, knees, bones, and Brain (*jian nao*).

(*cōng*) 聰
improves sharpness of the ears (hearing) (*cong er*).

Brightens (*míng*) 明
improves vision and benefits the eyes (*ming mu*).

Calms (*ān*) 安
quiets, calms, and pacifies the Spirit (*an shen*); calms the Fetus (*an tai*).

Clears
(*qīng*) 清
eliminates pathogenic influences such as Heat (*qing re*), Summerheat, and Fire; clears pathogenic influences and stagnation from the Brain (*qing nao*) to resolve mental disturbances.

(*tōng*) 通
moves obstructions and frees the nasal passages (*tong bi*).

Contains (*shè*) 舍
keeps the Blood within the vessels (prevents hemorrhaging) by strengthening the Qi function (*she xue*).

Cools (*liáng*) 涼
cools Heat in the Blood (*liang xue*).

Diffuses (xuān) 宣
circulates evenly, distributes, and disseminates Lung Qi *(xuan fei)*.

Dispels (qū) 祛
eliminates and dispels Wind *(qu feng)*, Wind-Heat, Wind-Cold, Wind-Dryness, Wind-Phlegm, and exterior Cold *(qu han)*.

Drains (xiè) 瀉
discharges and drains (downward) pathogenic influences of a specific Organ by way of the stool or urine: those of the Heart and Liver are drained through the urine; those of the Stomach and Lungs are drained through the stool.

Dries (zào) 燥
eliminates Dampness *(zao shi)* or Damp-Cold through the application of heat (moxibustion).

Enriches (zī) 滋
nourishes and tonifies the Yin *(zi yin)*.

Expands (kuān) 寬
frees, expands, and relaxes the chest *(kuan xiong)*.

Expedites (cuī) 催
promotes and stimulates lactation *(cui ru)* or labor *(cui chan)*.

Expels

(qū) 祛
expels parasites *(qu chong)*.

(pái) 排
dislodges and expels stones *(pai shi)* from the urinary tract or gallbladder.

Extinguishes (xī) 熄
pacifies the Liver and reduces Wind *(ping gan xi feng)*.

Facilitates (tōng) 通
facilitates and restores Qi flow *(tong qi)*, Blood flow *(tong xue)*, both Qi and Blood within the channels *(tong tiao qi xue)*; removes obstructions to normalize lactation *(tong ru zhi)*.

Generates (shēng) 生
promotes the production and increase of Fluids *(sheng jin)*.

Invigorates (húo) 活
activates, invigorates, and moves the Blood or Blood stasis *(huo xue)*.

Moistens (rùn) 潤
removes Dryness *(run zao)* by moistening the tissues and Organs; soothes and moistens the throat *(run hou)* and Intestines *(run chang)*.

Nourishes (yǎng) 養
supplements Blood and moistens Dryness *(yang xue run zao)*.

Opens (kāi) 開
clears obstructions and frees the passageways of the sensory orifices *(kai qiao)*, the ears *(kai er)*, and the eyes *(kai mu)*.

Promotes (lì) 利
stimulates and promotes urination *(li niao)*.

Raises (shēng) 昇
raises and strengthens the middle Qi *(sheng ti zhong qi)* characterized by prolapse, rectal bleeding, or chronic diarrhea due to Spleen, Yang, or Qi deficiency.

Redirects downward (jiàng) 降
redirects Qi downward (jiang ni qi) as in rebellious Stomach or Lung Qi and Liver Yang excess.

Reduces

(tuì) 退
reduces fever (tui re).

(xiāo) 消
resolves digestive stagnation (xiao dao) by improving digestion and removing food stagnation and abdominal masses.

Regulates (lǐ) 理 or (tiáo) 調
adjusts and regulates Organ imbalance (li wei), Qi (tiao qi), Blood (li xue), the middle Burner (li zhong), and menstruation (tiao jing); opens and regulates the Water Pathways or promotes fluid elimination including urination (tong tiao shui dao).

Relaxes (shū) 舒
soothes and relaxes the sinews (shu jin).

Releases (jiě) 解
relieves or releases the exterior (jie biao), usually by promoting sweating.

Resolves (lì) 利
discharges and resolves Dampness (li shi), Damp-Heat, and Damp-Summerheat by promoting urination.

Restores (huí) 回
restores balance to Yin and Yang (hui yang), especially in conditions of collapsed Yin or Yang.

Restrains (liǎn) 斂
holds back and restrains sweating (lian han).

Revives (xǐng) 醒
awakens or revives the Spirit (consciousness) (xing shen).

Softens (ruǎn) 軟
dissolves and softens hard masses (ruan jian san jie), as in goiter, scrofula, enlarged liver or spleen, and hard abdominal masses.

Spreads (shū) 疏
releases and disperses Liver Qi stagnation (shu gan).

Stabilizes (gù) 固
consolidates and secures Kidney Qi (gu shen se jing), Essence (gu jing), and the lower orifices (gu xia qiao).

Stimulates (fā) 發
stimulates and promotes sweating (fa han) in exterior conditions.

Strengthens (qiáng) 強
invigorates and restores strength to the sinews (qiang jin).

Subdues (qián) 潛
subdues and pacifies Liver Yang excess (qian yang).

Tonifies (bǔ) 補
strengthens, supplements, and vitalizes Organs (bu shen), Qi (bu qi), source Qi (bu yuan qi), protective Qi (bu wei qi), nutritive Qi (bu ying qi), Essence (bu jing), and Blood (bu xue).

Transforms *(huà)* 化
transforms Dampness *(hua shi)* including Damp-Heat, Damp-Summerheat, and Damp-Phlegm; transforms Phlegm *(hua tan)* including Phlegm-Cold, Dry-Phlegm, Phlegm-Heat, and Heart Phlegm.

Unblocks *(tōng)* 通
enlivens and invigorates the Blood vessels *(tong mai)* by restoring the Qi and Blood flow.

Warms *(wēn)* 温
invigorates and warms the Yang *(wen yang)* and interior Cold *(wen han)*.

CHAPTER 2

Point Classification

SOURCE POINTS
Yuán Xué

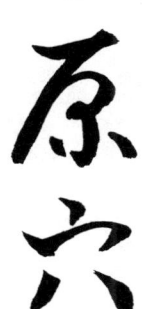

Each of the twelve channels has its own Source point which stores the corresponding Organ's source Qi. Source points are located in the vicinity of the wrists and ankles. Specifically, Yin channel Source points coincide with the Stream points, while Yang channel Source points are located immediately proximal to the Stream points.

Functions:
Produce an homeostatic effect on the corresponding Organs, regulating conditions of excess and deficiency.

Help to discern Organ disharmony when palpated.

Points:

Lung	L-9	(tai yuan)
Large Intestine	LI-4	(he gu)
Stomach	S-42	(chong yang)
Spleen	Sp-3	(tai bai)
Heart	H-7	(shen men)
Small Intestine	SI-4	(wan gu)
Bladder	B-64	(jing gu)
Kidney	K-3	(tai xi)
Pericardium	P-7	(da ling)
Triple Burner	TB-4	(yang chi)
Gallbladder	G-40	(qiu xu)
Liver	Liv-3	(tai chong)

CONNECTING POINTS
Luò Xué

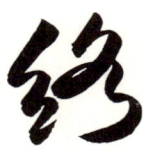
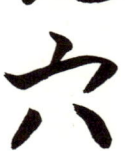

Connecting points bridge (by way of the connecting channels) the related Yin (internal) and Yang (external) channels of the corresponding phase (of the five phases). The fifteen Connecting points are comprised of a point for each of the twelve channels, the Conception and Governing vessels and a special Spleen point.

Functions:

Produce an homeostatic effect upon the corresponding Yin-Yang channels and Organs, primarily treating disharmonies between the two.

Converge with the Qi and Blood of the connecting channels and the lesser connecting channels, which provides a regulatory function over the entire system. Points particularly useful in serving this function include:

CV-15 *(jiu wei)*: regulates the Yin collaterals of the abdomen.

GV-1 *(chang qiang)*: regulates the Yang collaterals of the back and head.

Sp-21 *(da bao)*: regulates the Blood.

According to chapter 10 of the *Spiritual Axis (Ling shu)*, excess conditions due to rebellious Qi resulting in Blood flow disturbance may be treated by bloodletting at the affected channel's Connecting point.

Points:

Lung	L-7	(lie que)
Large Intestine	LI-6	(pian li)
Stomach	S-40	(feng long)
Spleen	Sp-4	(gong sun)
Heart	H-5	(tong li)
Small Intestine	SI-7	(zhi zheng)
Bladder	B-58	(fei yang)
Kidney	K-4	(da zhong)
Pericardium	P-6	(nei guan)
Triple Burner	TB-5	(wai guan)
Gallbladder	G-37	(guang ming)
Liver	Liv-5	(li gou)
Conception	CV-15	(jiu wei)
Governing	GV-1	(chang qiang)
Spleen (special)	Sp-21	(da bao)

NOTE: In clinical practice, Source and Connecting points are frequently used in combination with what is called the "guest-host method," where the "host" Source point of the channel primarily affected is used with the "guest" Connecting point of its related channel. This method restores harmony within a phase's Organs and channels. For channel or Organ deficiency, the Source point is tonified; for excess, it is sedated. The Connecting point of the related channel is then needled with an even method.

ALARM POINTS
Mù Xué

The channel Qi of each Organ converges at its Alarm point on the chest or abdomen. Not all of the Alarm points are located on the channel of the Organ which they affect.

Functions:

Treat the internal Organs and tonify the Yin (substantial) aspect.

Act as diagnostic reflex points which reveal an Organ's condition. Since the actual location of the reflex point can vary, the area around the point must also be palpated.

Points:

Lung	L-1	(zhong fu)
Large Intestine	S-25	(tian shu)
Stomach	CV-12	(zhong wan)
Spleen	Liv-13	(zhang men)
Heart	CV-14	(ju que)
Small Intestine	CV-4	(guan yuan)
Bladder	CV-3	(zhong ji)
Kidney	G-25	(jing men)
Pericardium	CV-17	(tan zhong)
Triple Burner	CV-5	(shi men)
Gallbladder	G-24	(ri yue)
Liver	Liv-14	(qi men)

ASSOCIATED POINTS
Bèi Shū Xué

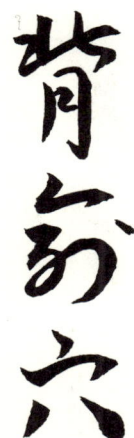

The channel Qi of each Organ converges at its Associated point on the body's posterior. These twelve points are located on the medial line of the Bladder channel.

Functions:

Treat the internal Organs, tonify the Yang (functional) aspect.

These points also treat the sensory organs and orifices corresponding to an internal Organ. For example, B-18, the Liver's Associated point, can treat eye disorders, the sensory organ related to that Organ.

Palpation of the point and the surrounding area can reveal the condition of an Organ as well as its related sensory organ or orifice.

Points:

Lung	B-13	(fei shu)
Large Intestine	B-25	(da chang shu)
Stomach	B-21	(wei shu)
Spleen	B-20	(pi shu)
Heart	B-15	(xin shu)
Small Intestine	B-27	(xiao chang shu)
Urinary Bladder	B-28	(pang guang shu)
Kidney	B-23	(shen shu)
Pericardium	B-14	(jue yin shu)
Triple Burner	B-22	(san jiao shu)
Gallbladder	B-19	(dan shu)
Liver	B-18	(gan shu)

NOTE: Alarm points are often used with Associated points for the treatment of diseased Organs requiring a stronger therapeutic effect.

ACCUMULATING POINTS
Xì Xué

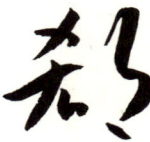
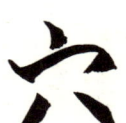

Accumulating points hold the channel's Qi and Blood in a deep hollow or crevice, which was traditionally viewed as the place where bone and flesh cross. These sixteen points are located on the twelve channels, the two Linking vessels and the two Heel vessels.

Functions:

Primarily treat acute-stage disorders, stubborn Organ disharmony and, in particular, excess conditions of both the channel and its corresponding Organ.

Used as diagnostic indicators of channel or Organ excess.

Points:

Lung	L-6	(kong zui)
Large Intestine	LI-7	(wen liu)
Stomach	S-34	(liang qiu)
Spleen	Sp-8	(di ji)
Heart	H-6	(yin xi)
Small Intestine	SI-6	(yang lao)
Bladder	B-63	(jin men)
Kidney	K-5	(shui quan)
Pericardium	P-4	(xi men)
Triple Burner	TB-7	(hui zong)
Gallbladder	G-36	(wai qiu)
Liver	Liv-6	(zhong du)
Yin-linking	K-9	(zhu bin)
Yang-linking	G-35	(yang jiao)
Yin-heel	K-8	(jiao xin)
Yang-heel	B-59	(fu yang)

FIVE TRANSPORTING POINTS
Wǔ Shū Xué

The Transporting points are five points located distal to the elbows and knees on each of the twelve channels. Their names describe the quality of the Qi flow likened to water along a channel's course. Each of the five types of points has specific therapeutic effects.

WELL
Jǐng 井

These points are located at the ends of the fingers and toes, where the channel Qi comes out of its source or well. They are used to treat "fullness below the heart" (*Classic of Difficulties*, chapter 68), which includes a stifling sensation in the chest, chest pain or mental illness.

Points:

Lung	L-11	(shao shang)
Large Intestine	LI-1	(shang yang)
Stomach	S-45	(li dui)
Spleen	Sp-1	(yin bai)
Heart	H-9	(shao chong)
Small Intestine	SI-1	(shao ze)
Bladder	B-67	(zhi yin)
Kidney	K-1	(yong quan)
Pericardium	P-9	(zhong chong)
Triple Burner	TB-1	(guan chong)
Gallbladder	G-44	(zu qiao yin)
Liver	Liv-1	(da dun)

POINT CLASSIFICATION

SPRING (or GUSHING)
Yíng 榮

These points are located primarily in the metacarpal and metatarsal regions, where the Qi flourishes and surfaces like water coming from a spring. They are used to treat "body heat" (febrile conditions) (*Classic of Difficulties*, chapter 68).

Points:

Lung	L-10	(yu ji)
Large Intestine	LI-2	(er jian)
Stomach	S-44	(nei ting)
Spleen	Sp-2	(da du)
Heart	H-8	(shao fu)
Small Intestine	SI-2	(qian gu)
Bladder	B-66	(zu tong gu)
Kidney	K-2	(ran gu)
Pericardium	P-8	(lao gong)
Triple Burner	TB-2	(ye men)
Gallbladder	G-43	(xia xi)
Liver	Liv-2	(xing jian)

STREAM (or TRANSPORTING)
Shū 輸

These points are located near or on the wrists and ankles, where the Qi flourishes and flows rapidly. They are used to treat "heavy body sensation and joint pain" (*Classic of Difficulties*, chapter 68) caused by painful obstruction or chronic disorders due to Damp-Heat.

Points:

Lung	L-9	(tai yuan)
Large Intestine	LI-3	(san jian)
Stomach	S-43	(xian gu)
Spleen	Sp-3	(tai bai)
Heart	H-7	(shen men)
Small Intestine	SI-3	(hou xi)
Bladder	B-65	(shu gu)
Kidney	K-3	(tai xi)
Pericardium	P-7	(da ling)
Triple Burner	TB-3	(zhong zhu)
Gallbladder	G-41	(zu lin qi)
Liver	Liv-3	(tai chong)

RIVER (or TRAVERSING)
Jīng 經

These points are located mainly on the forearm and lower leg, where the Qi becomes more abundant as it gains distance from its source. They are used to treat "alternate cold and heat as well as wheezing" (*Classic of Difficulties*, chapter 68), which includes throat problems, asthma and alternate fever and chills.

Points:

Lung	L-8	(jing qu)
Large Intestine	LI-5	(yang xi)
Stomach	S-41	(jie xi)
Spleen	Sp-5	(shang qiu)
Heart	H-4	(ling dao)
Small Intestine	SI-5	(yang gu)
Bladder	B-60	(kun lun)
Kidney	K-7	(fu liu)
Pericardium	P-5	(jian shi)

Triple Burner	TB-6	(zhi gou)
Gallbladder	G-38	(yang fu)
Liver	Liv-4	(zhong feng)

SEA (or UNITING)
Hé 合

These points are located at the elbows and knees, where the Qi is likened to the confluence of the river with the sea. They are used to treat "rebellious Qi as well as diarrhea" (*Classic of Difficulties*, chapter 68), which can lead to disorders of the Yang Organs, vomiting and irregular appetite.

Points:

Lung	L-5	(chi ze)
Large Intestine	LI-11	(qu chi)
Stomach	S-36	(zu san li)
Spleen	Sp-9	(yin ling quan)
Heart	H-3	(shao hai)
Small Intestine	SI-8	(xiao hai)
Bladder	B-40	(wei zhong)
Kidney	K-10	(yin gu)
Pericardium	P-3	(qu ze)
Triple Burner	TB-10	(tian jing)
Gallbladder	G-34	(yang ling quan)
Liver	Liv-8	(qu quan)

FIVE PHASE TRANSPORTING POINTS
Wǔ Xíng Shū Xué

These points correspond to the five phases:

	WELL	SPRING	STREAM	RIVER	SEA
Yin channel	wood	fire	earth	metal	water
Yang channel	metal	water	wood	fire	earth

There are various theories for the use of these points dating back to the *Classic of Difficulties*. Two of the most common are the mother-son method and the meridian treatment method, popular in Japanese acupuncture.

The mother-son method is based on the production cycle of the five phases, where certain points are used for tonification or sedation of their related channel or Organ. According to classical theory: the mother tonifies; the son sedates. For example, the mother (water) point for tonifying deficiency on the Liver channel (wood) is Liv-8 (*qu quan*). The son (fire) point for sedating excess is Liv-2 (*xing jian*).

The meridian treatment method treats excess or deficiency of an Organ or channel by using, in combination with the mother-son method, the phasic point (a point of the same phase as its corresponding channel and Organ) on the mother, son or controlling channels. For channel deficiency, first the mother point of the channel, then the phasic point of the mother channel are tonified. Finally, the phasic point of the controlling channel is sedated. For channel excess, first the controlling channel's phasic point is tonified, then the channel's son point and the phasic point of the son channel are sedated in succession. For example, Spleen deficiency is treated by tonifying the channel's mother point Sp-2 (*da du*), tonifying the Heart's phasic point H-8 (*shao fu*) and sedating the Liver's phasic point Liv-1 (*da dun*). For Spleen excess, first the Liver's phasic point Liv-1 (*da dun*) is tonified, then the Spleen's son point Sp-5 (*shang qiu*) and the Lung's phasic point L-8 (*jing qu*) are sedated.

Yin channels:

WOOD/ WELL	FIRE/ SPRING	EARTH/ STREAM	METAL/ RIVER	WATER/ SEA
L-11 (shao shang)	L-10 (yu ji)	L-9 (tai yuan)	L-8 (jing qu)	L-5 (chi ze)
Sp-1 (yin bai)	Sp-2 (da du)	Sp-3 (tai bai)	Sp-5 (shang qiu)	Sp-9 (yin ling quan)
H-9 (shao chong)	H-8 (shao fu)	H-7 (shen men)	H-4 (ling dao)	H-3 (shao hai)
K-1 (yong quan)	K-2 (ran gu)	K-3 (tai xi)	K-7 (fu liu)	K-10 (yin gu)
P-9 (zhong chong)	P-8 (lao gong)	P-7 (da ling)	P-5 (jian shi)	P-3 (qu ze)
Liv-1 (da dun)	Liv-2 (xing jian)	Liv-3 (tai chong)	Liv-4 (zhong feng)	Liv-8 (qu quan)

Yang channels:

METAL/ WELL	WATER/ SPRING	WOOD/ STREAM	FIRE/ RIVER	EARTH/ SEA
LI-1 (shang yang)	LI-2 (er jian)	LI-3 (san jian)	LI-5 (yang xi)	LI-11 (qu chi)
S-45 (li dui)	S-44 (nei ting)	S-43 (xian gu)	S-41 (jie xi)	S-36 (zu san li)
SI-1 (shao ze)	SI-2 (qian gu)	SI-3 (hou xi)	SI-5 (yang gu)	SI-8 (xiao hai)
B-67 (zhi yin)	B-66 (zu tong gu)	B-65 (shu gu)	B-60 (kun lun)	B-40 (wei zhong)
TB-1 (guan chong)	TB-2 (ye men)	TB-3 (zhong zhu)	TB-6 (zhi gou)	TB-10 (tian jing)
G-44 (zu qiao yin)	G-43 (xia xi)	G-41 (zu lin qi)	G-38 (yang fu)	G-34 (yang ling quan)

LOWER SEA (LOWER UNITING) POINTS
Xià Hé Xué

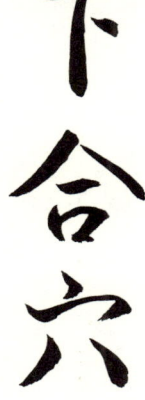

The six Lower Sea points, located on the lower extremities have, since ancient times, been connected with the Yang Organs, which are all located below the diaphragm. The Stomach, Bladder and Gallbladder Lower Sea points are located on their respective channels and are identical to the Sea points on these channels. The remaining three points are located on channels which have a similar energetic and physiologic function: the Small and Large Intestine Lower Sea points are on the Stomach channel, which controls digestion and downward movement of food and liquids; the Triple Burner Lower Sea point is on the Bladder channel, which controls water distribution and elimination.

Functions:
Very effective in treating Yang Organ disorders and often preferred to hand channel points.

Points:

Stomach	S-36	(zu san li)
Large Intestine	S-37	(shang ju xu)
Small Intestine	S-39	(xia ju xu)
Gallbladder	G-34	(yang ling quan)
Triple Burner	B-39	(wei yang)
Bladder	B-40	(wei zhong)

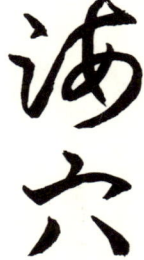

FOUR SEA POINTS
Sì Hǎi Xué

The Four Sea points are four groups of points that affect each of the "seas" and are described in the *Spiritual Axis* as "four seas into which the twelve channels flow." They are connected internally to the Organs, externally to the extremities. They act as reservoirs which are distinguished by the particular substance (Qi, Blood, Nourishment or Marrow) that they store.

Functions:
Regulate conditions of excess and deficiency within the seas. They are particularly useful when other significant symptoms are absent.

Points:

Sea of Qi
CV-17 (tan zhong)
 S-9   (ren ying)
GV-14 (da zhui)
GV-15 (ya men)

Associated Symptoms
Excess: sensation of fullness and heaviness in the chest, labored breathing, flushed face.

Deficiency: fatigue, difficulty in speaking with weak, slow and labored voice.

Sea of Blood
B-11   (da zhu)
S-37   (shang ju xu)
S-39   (xia ju xu)

Associated Symptoms
Excess: heavy body sensation, areas of stagnation with hard masses, pensiveness.

Deficiency: emaciation, chest tightness and discomfort, and apathy.

Sea of Nourishment
S-30   (qi chong)
S-36   (zu san li)

Associated Symptoms
Excess: abdominal distention.

Deficiency: hunger with no desire to eat.

Sea of Marrow
GV-16   (feng fu)
GV-20   (bai hui)

Associated Symptoms
Excess: increased vigor and sexual desire.

Deficiency: dizziness and vertigo, ringing in the ears, lassitude, desire to sleep, soreness and fatigue of the lower extremities.

NOTE: According to the *Spiritual Axis* (chapter 33), the extra points below each of the cervical spinous processes on the posterior midline between GV-14 (*da zhui*) and GV-15 (*ya men*) also affect the Sea of Qi; the Governing channel points between GV-16 (*feng fu*) and GV-20 (*bai hui*) can affect the Sea of Marrow.

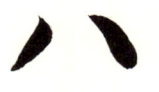
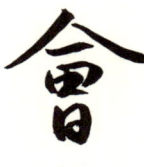

EIGHT INFLUENTIAL POINTS
Bā Huì Xué

The Influential points are those where the Qi and Essence of the eight types of tissues and substances converge.

Functions:
Disorders of a specific tissue or Organ can be treated by using the corresponding point.

Points:

Yin Organ	Liv-13	(zhang men)
Yang Organ	CV-12	(zhong wan)
Qi	CV-17	(tan zhong)
Blood	B-17	(ge shu)
Sinews	G-34	(yang ling quan)
Blood vessels	L-9	(tai yuan)
Bones	B-11	(da zhu)
Marrow	G-39	(xuan zhong)

EIGHT CONFLUENT POINTS
Bā Mài Jiāo Huì Xué

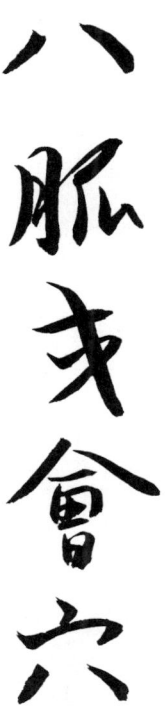

The eight miscellaneous vessels and the twelve channels intersect at the eight Confluent points located on the wrists and ankles. The miscellaneous vessels act as reservoirs for the twelve channels: they supplement the channels with Qi in times of deficiency and store the overflow of Qi in times of excess. These vessels are considered to be an "embryological" force which affects the psychic, protective, and structural aspects of the body.

Functions:

Regulate the eight miscellaneous vessels (see table below).

Maintain harmony and communication between the miscellaneous vessels and the twelve channels.

Affect specific body regions when used alone or in combination. The classical regions of influence represent a clinically useful application of these points (see table below).

Points:

Governing	SI-3	(hou xi)
Conception	L-7	(lie que)
Penetrating	Sp-4	(gong sun)
Girdle	G-41	(zu lin qi)
Yang-linking	TB-5	(wai guan)
Yin-linking	P-6	(nei guan)
Yang-heel	B-62	(shen mai)
Yin-heel	K-6	(zhao hai)

Vessel Disorders:
Key Symptoms and Regions of Influence

VESSEL	POINT	KEY SYMPTOMS	REGION OF INFLUENCE
Yin-linking	P-6	Chest pain	Heart, chest and stomach
Penetrating	Sp-4	Lower abdominal pain	
Governing	SI-3	Neck stiffness	Neck, shoulder, back and inner canthus
Yang-heel	B-62	Insomnia	
Yang-linking	TB-5	Alternate chills and fever	Neck, shoulder, cheek, back of ear, and outer canthus
Girdle	G-41	Lower back and loin weakness and pain	
Conception	L-7	Anterior midline pain	Chest, lungs, diaphragm and throat
Yin-heel	K-6	Excessive sleepiness	

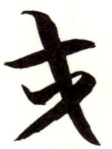
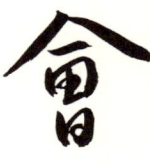
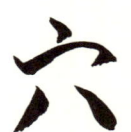

INTERSECTING POINTS
Jiāo Huì Xué

The points where two or more channels meet.

Functions:
Treat disturbances connected with the channel of origin (the channel or vessel to which the points belong) and disturbances of the intersecting channel or vessel.

CHAPTER 3

Point Images and Functions

L-1 (zhōng fŭ)
CENTRAL PALACE

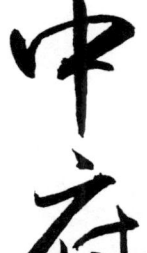

Alarm point of the Lungs and Intersecting point of the Spleen and Lung channel. Located below the acromial extremity of the clavicle, 1 unit inferior to the center of the infraclavicular fossa and 6 units lateral to the Conception vessel.

Image:
The name refers to this point's function as an administrative center for the Lungs which can indicate or affect an Organ's condition. Also, when *fu* appears with the flesh radical, it denotes the Yang Organs; when combined with *zhong* (central), it refers to this channel's internal origin in the Stomach within the middle Burner.

Functions:
Regulates and tonifies the Lungs (especially Qi and Yin), regulates the upper Burner, and tonifies ancestral Qi.
  Indications: pulmonary tuberculosis, pneumonia, Lung Abscess, asthma or bronchitis with cough and wheezing, edema due to Lung Qi deficiency, and dyspnea.
Diffuses Lung Qi, and expands and relaxes the chest:
  Indications: painful obstruction of the throat, chest fullness and pain, sore throat, and shoulder, neck and back pain.
Clears Heat (especially upper Burner):
  Indications: upper Burner-wasting and thirsting syndrome, fever with pulmonary symptoms, excessive sweating, and dry cough.

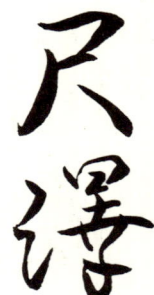

L-5 (chǐ zé)
CUBIT MARSH

Sea and Water point of the Lung channel.
With the elbow slightly flexed, located on the transverse cubital crease on the radial side of the tendon of the bicep brachii muscle.

Image:
Cubit indicates the distance from the middle position to the elbow crease; *marsh* refers to channel Qi flow which tends to slow down and spread out before continuing its course.

Functions:
Regulates and tonifies the Lungs (especially Yin and Qi), expands and relaxes the chest, and promotes redirection of rebellious Qi.

> Indications: childhood nutritional impairment, bronchitis, asthma, chest fullness and pain, vomiting, dyspnea, and neck and throat pain.

Clears Heat, dispels Wind-Heat and Wind-Dryness, moistens Dryness (especially Lung Dryness), and alleviates exterior conditions.

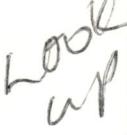

> Indications: upper Burner-wasting and thirsting syndrome, atrophy syndrome due to Lung Heat, erysipelas, psoriasis, cough due to Wind-Heat, afternoon fever due to Lung Yin deficiency, hemoptysis, dry cough, and sore throat.

Local effect: spasmodic elbow and arm pain.

Use moxibustion with caution.

L-6 (kŏng zuì)
EXTREME APERTURE

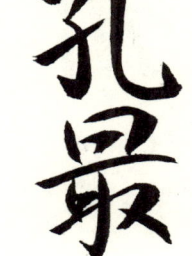

Accumulating point of the Lung channel.
Located 7 units superior to L-9 on a line connecting L-9 and L-5.

Image:
The name refers to this point's classification and location, where the channel Qi gathers and becomes excessive.

Functions:
Regulates the Lungs and redirects rebellious Qi downward.
  Indications: laryngitis, tonsillitis, bronchiecstasis, asthma, cough, sore throat, epigastric pain, and headache.
Clears Heat and Heat in the Blood and stimulates sweating.
  Indications: pulmonary tuberculosis, hemoptysis, fever without sweating, and hemorrhoids.

Local effect: pain and motor impairment of the elbow and arm.

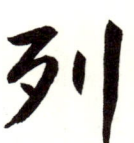
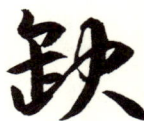

L-7 (liè quē)
BROKEN SEQUENCE

Connecting point of the Lung channel and Confluent point of the Conception vessel.
Located in the slight depression at the origin of the styloid process of the radius 1.5 units proximal to the wrist crease (L-9).

Image:
The name suggests an interruption in Qi flow where the Connecting channel begins. Also, a classical meaning for *lie que* refers to the strong reaction and propagation of Qi that occurs with needling of this point.

Functions:
Regulates the Lungs (especially Qi).
   Indications: asthma, tonsillitis, bronchitis with cough, nasal discharge, productive cough, sore throat, and frontal and lateral headache.
Diffuses Lung Qi, stimulates sweating, dispels Wind-Cold,△ Wind-Heat and Cold,△ and transforms Phlegm-Cold△ and Damp-Phlegm.
   Indications: common cold, rhinitis, urticaria, facial paralysis, hemiplegia, deviation of mouth and eyes, lockjaw, stiff neck, and toothache.
Regulates the Conception vessel.
   Indications: burning sensation during urination, chills, pain and itching along anterior midline of the abdomen and chest, pain and inflammation of the umbilicus, penile pain, and redness, swelling and pain along the sternum.
Local effect: wrist weakness.

L-8 (jīng qú)
PASSING DITCH

River and Metal point of the Lung channel.
Located in the depression on the radial side of the radial artery 1 unit proximal to the wrist crease (L-9).

Image:
The name refers to this point's location on the channel where the Qi flow passes through a slight depression or ditch proximal to the wrist crease.

Functions:
Regulates the Lungs, and expands and relaxes the chest.
   Indications: asthma, cough, chest pain with vomiting, chest pain radiating to the upper back, esophageal spasm or pain, sore throat, and dyspnea.

Local effect: wrist pain.

Moxibustion is contraindicated.

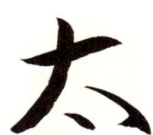

L-9 (tài yuān)
GREAT ABYSS

Stream, Source, and Earth point of the Lung channel and Influential point of the Blood vessels.
Located in the depression at the radial side of the radial artery at the transverse wrist crease.

Image:
The name refers to the Qi which dives deeply into the interior like a waterfall. This image perhaps also refers to the area just distal to this point, where the pulse disappears as the course of the artery runs internally.

Functions:
Regulates and tonifies the Lungs (especially Yin and Qi), enriches Yin, clears Heat, moistens Dryness, transforms Phlegm-Heat, Damp-Phlegm and Dry-Phlegm (especially upper Burner), and promotes redirection of rebellious Qi.
>Indications: pulmonary tuberculosis, bronchitis, Lung Abscess, pertussis, chronic cough and asthma due to Yin deficiency, chest pain, palpitations, irritability and agitation, and sensation of heat in the palms.

Unblocks the pulses and opens the sensory orifices.
>Indications: heatstroke, coma, and various conditions with a collapsed pulse.

Local effect: wrist pain and weakness.

MOST IMP. PT. TO TONIFY LUNG QI & YIN

"Qi is commander of blood
AIR & FOOD = Qi - HARMONIZES gathering Qi & BLOOD

L-10 (yú jì)
FISH BORDER

Spring and Fire point of the Lung channel.
Located on the radial border at the midpoint of the first metacarpal bone at the junction of the red and white skin.

Image:
The name refers to the thenar eminence which resembles the abdomen of a fish. *Border* indicates where the Lung channel traverses the radial border of the thenar eminence.

Functions:
Regulates the Lungs, clears Lung Fire and Heat and cools Heat in the Blood, dispels Wind-Heat, and stimulates sweating.
  Indications: upper Burner-wasting and thirsting syndrome, pneumonia, asthma, fever or tidal fever, emotional distress, mastitis, chest and back pain, hemoptysis, and headache.
Moistens the throat.
  Indications: sore throat, hoarseness, voice loss, throat pain, dryness, redness or swelling, tonsillitis, and dyspnea.

↑ Lu HEAT AGITATES HT ∴ emotional distress

L-11 (shào shāng)
LESSER METAL'S NOTE

Well and Wood point of the Lung channel.
Located about 0.1 unit from the radial corner of the thumbnail.

Image:
The name refers to the reduced amount of Qi at the distal end of the extremity and channel. *Shang* is the second note in the ancient Chinese musical scale and, like this point's corresponding channel and Organ, is associated with the metal phase.

Functions:
Regulates the Lungs, clears Lung Fire, Heat and Summerheat, and dispels Wind-Heat.
> Indications: upper Burner-wasting and thirsting syndrome, febrile diseases, asthma, pneumonia, cough due to Lung Heat, vomiting or fullness of the epigastric region due to Summerheat, epistaxis, and chest pain with excessive sweating.

Moistens the throat.
> Indications: tonsillitis, mumps, throat pain, dryness, redness or swelling.

Revives consciousness, calms the Spirit, and restores collapsed Yang.
> Indications: Wind-stroke, collapsing syndrome, seizures, heatstroke, hysteria, coma, delirium, and disorientation.

Local effect: finger pain and contracture.

LI-1 *(shāng yáng)*
METAL'S NOTE YANG

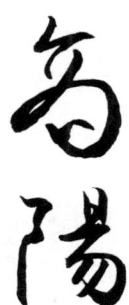

Well and Metal point of the Large Intestine channel. Located about 0.1 unit from the radial corner of the second fingernail.

Image:
Metal's Note Yang begins the Large Intestine channel, the Yang channel of the metal phase, and corresponds to metal of the Five Phase Transporting point classification. *Shang* suggests the musical note that corresponds to metal.

Functions:
Diffuses Lung Qi, dispels Wind-Heat, and clears Lung Fire and Heat.°
  Indications: febrile diseases, asthma, tinnitus, deafness, cough with chest fullness, common cold with high fever and sweating, upper jaw toothache, and cough with shoulder pain radiating to the supraclavicular fossa.

Moistens the throat.
  Indications: mumps, tonsillitis, sore throat, submandibular swelling, and dry mouth.

Revives consciousness.
  Indications: collapsing syndrome, Wind-stroke, and coma.

Local effect: finger numbness.

Use moxibustion with caution.

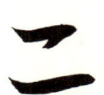
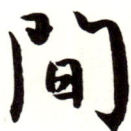

LI-2 (èr jiān)
SECOND INTERVAL

Spring and Water point of the Large Intestine channel.

With the finger slightly flexed, located on the radial side of the second finger distal to the metacarpophalangeal joint at the junction of the red and white skin.

Image:
The name indicates this point's position as the second point of the Large Intestine channel.

Functions:
Dispels Wind-Heat and clears Heat.
> Indications: hemiplegia, facial paralysis, trigeminal neuralgia, fever, somnolence, toothache, headache, blurred vision, epistaxis, and shoulder and back pain.

Moistens the throat.
> Indications: tonsillitis, sore throat, dry mouth, submandibular swelling, and esophageal spasms.

LI-3 (sān jiān)
THIRD INTERVAL

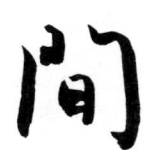

Stream and Wood point of the Large Intestine channel.

While making a loose fist, located on the radial side of the second finger in the depression proximal to the head of the second metacarpal bone.

Image:
The name indicates this point's position as the third point on the Large Intestine channel.

Functions:
Regulates the Large Intestine, clears Heat, and transforms Damp-Heat.

> Indications: malarial disorders, trigeminal neuralgia, somnolence, conjunctivitis, eye redness, swelling and pain, toothache, abdominal distention, dyspnea, borborygmus, diarrhea, and constipation due to excess Heat.

Moistens the throat.

> Indications: tonsillitis, painful obstruction of the throat with excessive mucus, sore throat, and mouth and lip dryness.

Local effect: redness and swelling of the fingers and the dorsum of the hand.

LI-4 *(hé gǔ)*
ADJOINING VALLEYS

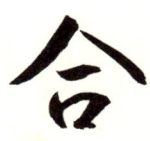

Source point of the Large Intestine channel.
Located on the back of the hand, halfway between the junction of the first and second metacarpal bones and about 0.5 unit above the margin of the web.

Image:
The name refers to this point's location between the first and second metacarpals which form a depression or *valley* when the thumb is abducted.

Functions:
Alleviates exterior conditions, promotes or restrains sweating, reduces fever, facilitates Qi flow, dispels Wind, Wind-Cold, Wind-Dryness, Wind-Heat and Cold, clears Fire and Heat, moistens Dryness, transforms Damp-Heat, Phlegm, Damp-Phlegm, Phlegm-Cold△ and Dry-Phlegm, generates Fluids, regulates and tonifies Qi, tonifies protective Qi, and alleviates pain.

> Indications: atrophy syndrome of the upper body, infantile paralysis, childhood nutritional impairment, upper Burner-wasting and thirsting syndrome, Hot painful obstruction, trigeminal neuralgia due to Wind-Heat, eczema or erysipelas due to Wind-Heat, Qi-type painful urinary dysfunction, common cold, mumps, amenorrhea, voice loss, otitis media, urticaria, hemiplegia, fever without sweating, fever and chills, toothache, facial paralysis or swelling, sneezing, eye redness, pain and swelling, and frontal headache.

Regulates the Lungs (especially Qi) and drains pathogenic influences from the Lungs.

Indications: pertussis, asthma, bronchitis, common cold with thirst.

Regulates and moistens the Large Intestine.
Indications: dysenteric disorders, infantile diarrhea, appendicitis with fever, constipation or diarrhea due to Heat, and abdominal pain.

Softens hard masses.
Indications: lymphangitis, goiter, scrofula, and furuncles.

Relaxes the sinews.
Indications: closed-type Wind-stroke, muscular tetany with lockjaw, hysteria, and facial pain and paralysis.

Moistens the throat and benefits the tongue.
Indications: tonsillitis, painful obstruction of the throat, mumps, voice loss, and tongue stiffness and pain.

Restores collapsed Yang, clears Summerheat, and opens the sensory orifices.
Indications: closed or abandoned-type coma, collapsing syndrome, heatstroke, and fever due to Summerheat.

Opens and brightens the eyes.
Indications: all eye disorders including glaucomatous disorders, strabismus, conjunctivitis, myopia, blurred vision, and sudden blindness.

Expedites labor.
Indications: aids the aborting of a dead fetus and delayed or difficult labor.

Clears the nose.
Indications: all nasal disorders including rhinitis, epistaxis, sinusitis, and rhinorrhea.

Local effect: lockjaw, arm pain and swelling, and contracture or paralysis of the fingers.

Needling contraindicated during pregnancy.

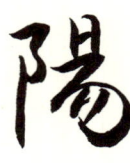
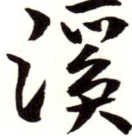

LI-5 (yáng xī)
YANG STREAM

River and Fire point of the Large Intestine channel.

Located on the wrist in the depression between the tendons of the extensor pollicis longus and brevis muscles.

Image:
The name refers to this point's location in a stream-like depression between two tendons on the wrist where the channel Qi is vital and intense like a mountain stream.

Functions:
Dispels Wind-Heat, clears Heat, and transforms Damp-Heat.
> Indications: various skin disorders with itching including eczema and urticaria, toothache, sore throat, headache, eye redness, swelling and pain, hearing loss, tinnitus, tongue root pain, fever with chest pain, and spasms in the back.

Calms the Spirit.
> Indications: febrile diseases with restlessness, seizures, and mania.

Local effect: wrist pain or swelling.

LI-6 *(piān lì)*
DEVIATED PASSAGE

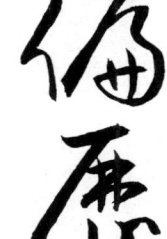

Connecting point of the Large Intestine channel.

Located 3 units proximal to LI-5 on a line connecting LI-5 and LI-11.

Image:
The name suggests that this is the point from which the channel Qi is redirected into the Connecting channel.

Functions:
Clears Heat, moistens Dryness, and dispels Wind.
  Indications: seizures, facial paralysis, facial and upper body edema, conjunctivitis, dim vision, deviation of mouth, constipation due to excess Heat, epistaxis, and urinary retention.

Moistens the throat.
  Indications: tonsillitis, throat dryness, soreness and numbness.

Local effect: hand and arm pain and aches.

LI-7 *(wēn liū)*
TEMPERATE FLOW

Accumulating point of the Large Intestine channel. Located halfway between LI-5 and LI-11.

Image:
The name indicates this point's classification as an Accumulating point and its ability to balance and soften the flow of channel Qi.

Functions:
Regulates the Large Intestine, clears Heat, and transforms Dampness.
> Indications: stomatitis, abdominal pain and distention, borborygmus, belching, epistaxis, headache with fever, facial edema, swelling, and heaviness of the extremities.

Moistens the throat and benefits the tongue.
> Indications: protruded tongue, sore throat, mouth and tongue swelling, pain and inflammation, and sore throat.

Local effect: shoulder and arm ache.

LI-10 *(shŏu sān lǐ)*
ARM THREE MILES

Located 2 units distal to LI-11 on a line connecting LI-5 and LI-11.

Image:
The name suggests this point's ability to build up physical strength and endurance. *Shou san li* literally means "three units on the arm," referring to its location three units below the bony protuberance of the epicondyle (see S-36 *[zu san li]*).

Functions:
Regulates the Stomach and Intestines and reduces digestive stagnation.

Indications: facial paralysis, arm paralysis after stroke, arm cramps, arm edema, shoulder pain and hemiplegia, swollen jaw, abdominal distention, stomachache, indigestion, fecal incontinence, diarrhea and/or vomiting, toothache, and voice loss.

Softens hard masses.

Indications: goiter, breast abscess, and swelling in the submandibular region.

Local effect: upper arm numbness and pain, muscle spasms causing inability to extend elbow and atrophy of the wrist extensor muscles.

LI-11 *(qū chí)*

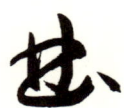
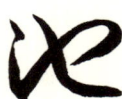

CROOKED POOL

Sea and Earth point of the Large Intestine channel.
With the elbow flexed, located in the depression at the lateral end of the transverse cubital crease.

Image:
Crooked, like a bend in a river, refers to this point's location at the bend of the elbow in the crease. Like the Sea points, *pool* refers to the flow of Qi as it slows down and spreads out.

Functions:
Alleviates exterior conditions, dispels Wind, Wind-Heat and Wind-Dryness, reduces fever, clears Fire, Heat, Summerheat and cools Heat in the Blood, moistens Dryness, stimulates sweating, transforms Damp-Heat and Damp-Summerheat, invigorates the Blood, and facilitates Qi and Blood flow.

Indications: Wind-stroke, febrile diseases, malarial disorders, Qi-type painful urinary dysfunction, Hot painful obstruction, common cold due to Wind-Heat, hypertension due to Yang excess, atrophy syndrome of the upper body, scabies, erysipelas, urticaria or eczema due to Wind-Heat, all skin disorders due to Heat in the Blood or Damp-Heat, herpes zoster, infantile paralysis, psoriasis, measles, mumps, allergies, anemia, heatstroke, convulsions, bronchitis, hemiplegia, upper extremity edema, acute lower back pain, deficient menstruation, menopausal hot flush, lassitude and depression, blurred vision, painful obstruction of the throat with swelling, and toothache.

Regulates and moistens the Large Intestine.

Indications: Intestinal Abscess, appendicitis or acute diarrhea with fever, constipation, and abdominal pain and distention.

Regulates the Lungs (especially Qi) and drains pathogenic influences from the Lungs.

Indications: bronchitis and chest fullness and pain.

Softens hard masses.

Indications: goiter, scrofula, boils, and carbuncles.

Benefits the shoulders.

Indications: shoulder pain, stiffness, and motor impairment.

Local effect: elbow and arm pain, swelling or motor impairment.

LI-14 (bì nào)
UPPER ARM'S MUSCULATURE

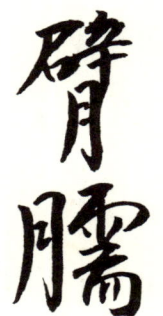

Intersecting point of the Yang-linking vessel on the Large Intestine channel.

Located on the lower border of the deltoid muscle and the radial side of the humerus, approximately 3 units below LI-15.

Image:
The name refers to the point's anatomical location and the areas it affects.

Functions:
Dispels Wind and Wind-Heat and relaxes the sinews.
> Indications: painful obstruction of the throat, arm and shoulder pain, upper limb paralysis, and neck stiffness.

Brightens the eyes.
> Indications: various eye disorders including conjunctivitis and myopia.

LI-15 *(jiān yú)*
SHOULDER'S CORNER

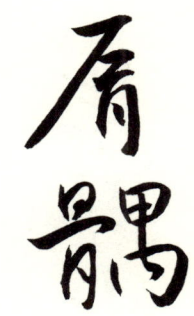

Intersecting point of the Yang-heel vessel on the Large Intestine channel.

Located directly inferior to the anterior border of the acromion where a depression is formed when the arm is abducted.

Image:
The name refers to this point's location and to its influence upon the shoulder articulations.

Functions:
Relaxes the sinews, benefits the shoulders, and dispels Wind and clears Heat.

> Indications: atrophy syndrome of the upper body, hypertension, urticaria due to Wind-Heat, hemiplegia, shoulder bursitis or painful obstruction, shoulder pain, stiffness and inflammation, shoulder, arm or hand paralysis, muscular spasms, and excessive sweating.

Softens hard masses.

> Indications: goiter and scrofula.

LI-16 *(jù gǔ)*
GIANT BONE

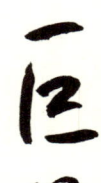
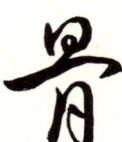

Intersecting point of the Yang-heel vessel on the Large Intestine channel.

Located in the depression about 1 unit medial to the acromioclavicular joint.

Image:
The name is a classical term for the clavicle bone and also refers to the general area this point affects, including the various large bones that form the shoulder girdle.

Functions:
Benefits the shoulders.

> Indications: childhood nutritional impairment, painful obstruction of the shoulder, shoulder and upper extremity pain, inflammation and motor impairment, and cough.

Softens hard masses.

> Indications: goiter and scrofula.

LI-18 *(fú tū)*
RELIEVE PROMINENCE

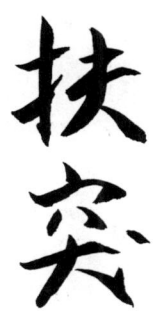

Level with the laryngeal prominence, located just between the two heads of the sternocleidomastoid muscle.

Image:
The name refers to this point's proximity to, and its ability to aid the laryngeal prominence or Adam's apple. *Fu* literally means "four fingers' breadth," which is the approximate distance of the point from the laryngeal prominence.

Functions:
Moistens the throat, diffuses Lung Qi, and transforms Phlegm.
> Indications: various throat or neck problems including cough, sore or dry throat, asthmatic wheezing, excessive throat and chest mucus and difficulty in swallowing, aphasia, and dyspnea.

Softens hard masses.
> Indications: goiter and scrofula.

LI-20 *(yíng xiāng)*
RECEIVING FRAGRANCE

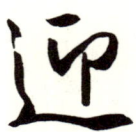
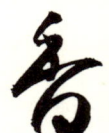

Intersecting point of Stomach and Large Intestine channels.

Located on the nasolabial sulcus, level with the midpoint of the lateral border of the ala nasi.

Image:
The name refers to this point's anatomical location next to the nasal orifice and its effect on the olfactory function. Also, *fragrance* refers to the channel (Stomach) that this point intersects and its correspondence to the earth phase.

Functions:
Clears the nose, dispels Wind, Wind-Cold and Wind-Heat, and clears Heat.

> Indications: various skin disorders of the face including eczema, acne, trigeminal neuralgia, facial itching and swelling and swollen or cracked lips, common cold with nasal obstruction, rhinitis, sinusitis, nasal polyps, epistaxis, and diminished sense of smell.

Use moxibustion with caution.

S-1 *(chéng qì)*
CONTAIN TEARS

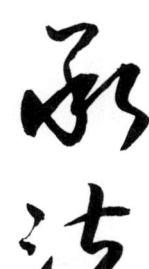

Intersecting point of the Conception and Yang-heel vessels on the Stomach channel.

Located directly inferior to the pupil on the inferior ridge of the orbital cavity.

Image:
The name refers to this point's anatomical location, the lower eyelid, which stores and releases tears.

Functions:
Brightens the eyes, dispels Wind and clears Heat.
   Indications: all eye disorders including excessive tearing due to Wind, myopia, conjunctivitis and eye pain, redness and swelling.

Moxibustion is contraindicated.

S-2 (sì bái)
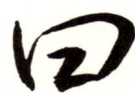
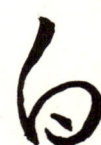
FOUR BRIGHTNESS

Located directly inferior to the pupil on the inferior ridge of the orbital cavity.

Image:
The name refers to this point's function of brightening the eyes, enabling one to see into the "four directions" with renewed clarity.

Functions:
Brightens the eyes, dispels Wind and Cold, clears Heat, and relaxes the sinews (especially facial).

    Indications: all eye problems including hyperthyroidism with protruding eyes, trigeminal neuralgia, color blindness, conjunctivitis, eyelid spasm, facial pain or paralysis, eye redness, soreness and itching.

Expels parasites.

    Indications: roundworm in bile duct and intestinal parasites.

Clears the nose.

    Indications: rhinitis, sinus headache, sinusitis, and allergic facial swelling.

Use moxibustion with caution.

S-3 (jù liáo)
LARGE OPENING

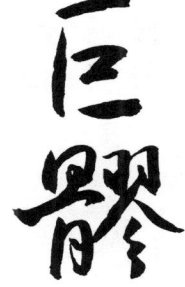

Intersecting point of the Yang-heel vessel on the Stomach channel.

Located directly inferior to S-1 at the level of the inferior border of the ala nasi.

Image:
The name refers to this point's anatomical location at the edge of the maxillary canine fossa as the maxilla curves posteriorly and laterally, where there appears to be an opening or space formed between the maxilla and the ramus of the mandible.

Functions:
Dispels Wind and Cold△ and relaxes the sinews (especially facial).
    Indications: facial paralysis, trigeminal neuralgia, cheek and lip pain and swelling, eyelid spasm and toothache.

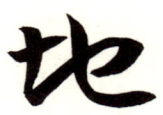
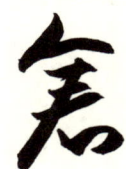

S-4 (dì cāng)
EARTH GRANARY

Intersecting point of the Large Intestine channel and the Yang-heel vessel on the Stomach channel.

Located 0.4 unit lateral to the corner of the mouth.

Image:
The name refers to this point's "topographic" location, the mouth, which is the orifice that corresponds to the Spleen and Stomach of the earth phase. Food is ingested, assimilated and secreted and a portion is stored in the form of Qi and Essence for times of need.

Functions:
Dispels Wind and Cold and relaxes the sinews (especially facial).

> Indications: facial paralysis, trigeminal neuralgia, excessive salivation, eyelid spasm, deviation of the mouth, inability to close the mouth, cold sores on the lips, lip spasms, toothache, and swollen cheeks.

S-6 (jiá chē)
JAW VEHICLE

With the teeth slightly clenched, at the prominence of the masseter muscle at the lateral aspect of the lower mandible, about 1 unit anterosuperior to the mandibular angle.

Image:
The name refers to this point's location in the masseter muscle which promotes movement of the jaw.

Functions:
Moistens the throat, dispels Wind and Cold△ and clears Heat.

    Indications: mumps, facial paralysis, neck pain and stiffness, sore throat, voice loss, and toothache.

Relaxes the sinews.

    Indications: temporomandibular joint arthritis or dysfunction and lockjaw.

S-7 (xià guān)
LOWER HINGE

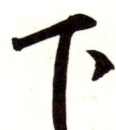
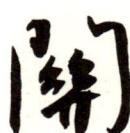

Intersecting point of the Gallbladder channel on the Stomach channel.

With the mouth slightly open, located in the depression at the inferior border of the zygomatic arch anterior to the condyloid process.

Image:
The name refers to this point's anatomical location and area of influence at the temporomandibular articulation.

Functions:

Dispels Wind, Cold△ and Wind-Heat, and clears Heat.
> Indications: temporomandibular joint arthritis or dysfunction, trigeminal neuralgia, facial paralysis, lockjaw, gingivitis, and toothache.

Opens the ears.
> Indications: deafness, tinnitus, otitis media, and earache.

S-8 (tóu wéi)
SKULL'S SAFEGUARD

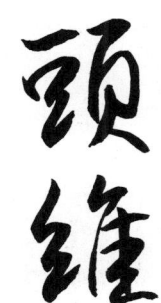

Intersecting point of the Gallbladder channel and the Yang-linking vessel on the Stomach channel.

Located at the angle of the forehead, 4.5 units lateral to the midline of the head on the coronal suture.

Image:
The name is a figurative reference to the point's location on the coronal suture. *Wei* means "to tie up," safeguard, preserve and support like a suture. It is also said to be the place where the Chinese of ancient times fastened their hats.

Functions:
Dispels Wind and clears Heat.
  Indications: cerebral congestion, frontal headache, dizziness and vertigo, and facial pain.

Brightens the eyes.
  Indications: excessive tearing due to Wind, blurred vision, and eyelid spasms.

Use moxibustion with caution.

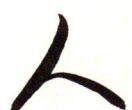
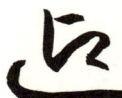

S-9 (rén yíng)
MAN'S WELCOME

Sea of Qi point, Intersecting point of the Gallbladder channel on the Stomach channel.

Level with the laryngeal prominence, located on the anterior border of the sternocleidomastoid muscle where the pulse of the common carotid artery can be felt.

Image:
The name refers to this point's position on the Stomach channel, where the channel Qi descends from the neck into the mid-body zone between the lower part of the neck and the chest. In addition, ancient Chinese philosophers associated this body zone with man in the triad of heaven, man, and earth.

Functions:
Diffuses Lung Qi, regulates Qi.

    Indications: asthma, high or low blood pressure, dyspnea, vomiting, diarrhea and vomiting, and headache.

Moistens the throat.

    Indications: esophageal constriction with inability to swallow, speech impairment, sore throat, swollen larynx, and painful obstruction of the throat.

Softens hard masses.

    Indications: goiter and scrofula.

CAUTION: *avoid puncturing artery. Moxibustion is contraindicated.*

S-18 (rŭ gēn)
BREAST ROOT

Located in the fifth intercostal space directly below the nipple, 4 units lateral to the Conception vessel.

Image:
The name refers to this point's location at the base of the breast.

Functions:
Diffuses Lung Qi, expands and relaxes the chest.
> Indications: chest and hypochondriac fullness and pain, stifling sensation in the chest, cough, bronchitis, and asthma.

Expedites and facilitates lactation.
> Indications: insufficient lactation and mastitis.

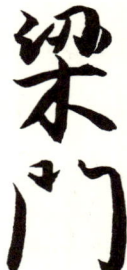

S-21 *(liáng mén)*
CONNECTING GATE

Located 2 units lateral to CV-12, 4 units above the umbilicus.

Image:
The name refers to this point's role in harmonizing and regulating the Organs of the middle Burner. *Liang*, with the grain radical, also means "millet" and suggests a relationship with the primary digestive Organs (Spleen and Stomach) and the Stomach's internal anatomical opening, the cardia *(ben men)* or "gate" that receives grain or foodstuffs.

Functions:
Regulates and strengthens the Spleen (especially Yang), Stomach (especially Qi) and middle Burner, clears middle Burner Heat and reduces digestive stagnation.

> Indications: abdominal or hypochondriac pain due to Qi stagnation, stomach and duodenal ulcers, acute and chronic gastritis, epigastric pain, chronic loose stools or diarrhea, undigested food in stool, indigestion, and poor appetite.

Raises middle Qi.

> Indications: prolapse of the Stomach.

S-25 (tiān shū)
HEAVEN'S AXIS

Alarm point of the the Large Intestine.

Located 2 units lateral to the center of the umbilicus, CV-8.

Image:
The name refers to this point's location and area of influence. This point is located level with the umbilicus and CV-8 or "Spirit's Palace Gate," the entry gate for the Spirit and hereditary energies (source Qi, Essence, ancestral Qi, etc.) which are connected with the prenatal stage of human development. *Tian shu* is also an ancient name for a star in the constellation Ursa Minor, which was viewed as a pole star until its passage through the procession of equinoxes moved it away from the true pole. This suggests the point's location slightly off-center from the umbilicus.

Functions:
Regulates the Spleen (especially Qi and Yang), the Stomach (especially Qi and Yin) and the middle and lower Burners, moistens and regulates the Intestines, generates Fluids, tonifies nutritive Qi, reduces digestive stagnation, clears (abdominal) Heat, transforms (Intestinal) Dampness and Damp-Heat, dries Dampness and Damp-Cold,△ warms Cold,△ and regulates Qi and Blood.

> Indications: Intestinal Abscess, dysenteric disorders with or without bleeding, hernia, acute intestinal obstruction, abdominal masses, stomach and duodenal ulcers, colitis, enteritis, appendicitis, pancreatitis, borborygmus, indigestion, vomiting, diarrhea, abdominal pain and distention, constipation due to Heat, loose stool due to pulmonary tuberculosis, infantile diarrhea, periumbilical pain, and edema.

Regulates menstruation.
> Indications: infertility, endometriosis, irregular menstruation, dysmenorrhea, and leukorrhea with blood.

Expels parasites and urinary tract stones.
> Indications: intestinal parasites and stones lodged in the upper urinary tract.

Needling contraindicated during pregnancy.

S-28 (shuĭ dào)
WATERWAY

Located 2 units lateral to CV-4, 3 units below the umbilicus.

Image:
The name refers to this point's control over and location near (in the deep internal position) the ureter, which conveys urine or fluid wastes.

Functions:
Regulates the Water Pathways and Bladder, and transforms Damp-Heat (especially lower Burner).

    Indications: painful urinary dysfunction, acute nephritis, dymenorrhea and leukorrhea, ascites, edema, lower abdominal distention, urinary retention, lower back pain, orchitis, and pain radiating to the genital region.

Expels (urinary tract) stones.

    Indications: Kidney stones lodged in the upper and lower tract.

S-29 *(guī lái)*
RETURN

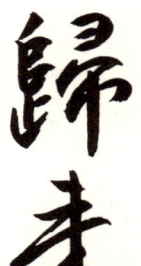

Located 2 units lateral to CV-3, 4 units below the umbilicus.

Image:
The name refers to this point's influence on the menstrual cycle and its ability to restore the tissue and position of the uterus to normal.

Functions:
Regulates menstruation, tranforms (lower Burner) Damp-Heat, warms (lower Burner) Cold,^△ and raises middle Qi.

> Indications: hernial disorders due to Cold, impotence and infertility, endometriosis, irregular menstruation, dysmenorrhea, amenorrhea, leukorrhea, uterine prolapse, adnexal inflammation, vaginitis, scrotal and urethral pain, orchitis, prostatitis, and lower abdominal pain and cold.

S-30 *(qì chōng)*
QI'S BREAKTHROUGH

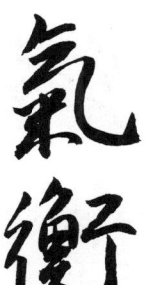

Sea of Nourishment point, Intersecting point of the Conception, Governing and Penetrating vessels on the Stomach channel.

Located 2 units lateral to CV-2 on the superior ridge of the pubic tubercle.

Image:
The name refers to the deep-lying Qi of the Stomach channel and the various vessels that intersect, gather and surface from the body's interior. *Chong* is the name for the Penetrating vessel, which begins its external pathway at this point.

Functions:
Stabilizes the Essence and the lower orifices, regulates Qi and Blood, tonifies nutritive Qi, regulates menstruation and the Penetrating vessel, invigorates and contains the Blood.

> Indications: infertility and impotence, spermatorrhea, irregular menstruation, dysmenorrhea due to Blood stasis, uterine tumors or fibroids, uterine hemorrhage, uterus failing to return to normal shape after childbirth, urethral, testicle or penile pain, kidney pain and swelling, pain of the external genitalia, lower abdominal pain, swelling and cold, and hunger with no desire to eat due to deficiency.

Raises middle Qi.
> Indications: hernial disorders and uterovaginal prolapse.

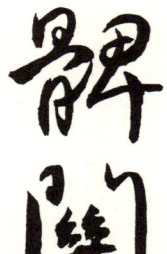

S-31 *(bì guān)*
HIP'S BORDER GATE

Located directly below the anterior superior iliac spine, level with the lower border of the pubic symphysis.

Image:
The name refers to this point's location near and influence on the border of the lower extremity and the trunk at the hip. It also refers to its function of controlling Qi going into the leg.

Functions:
Benefits the hips, dispels Wind and Cold,[△] clears Heat, facilitates Qi and Blood flow, and transforms Dampness.

> Indications: lower extremity atrophy syndrome, inguinal lymphadenitis or hernia, painful obstruction or heaviness of the lower extremities, restricted movement of the hip due to atrophy or paralysis, leg pain, blocked arterial circulation into the leg, lower back pain radiating to the medial aspect of the leg, and lower extremity weakness.

S-32 (fú tù)
PROSTRATE RABBIT

Located 6 units above the lateral superior border of the patella on the line connecting the anterior superior iliac spine and the lateral border of the patella.

Image:
This point is just lateral to the rectus femoris muscle, which resembles a rabbit lying prone.

Functions:
Dispels Wind and Cold,△ clears Heat, and transforms Dampness.

> Indications: painful obstruction of the knee, sensation of heaviness of the head, leg Qi, paralysis of the extensor muscles of the knee, urticaria, hemiplegia and abdominal distention, pain and cold of the lower back, thigh and knee.

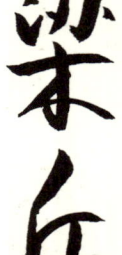

S-34 *(liáng qiū)*
CONNECTING MOUND

Accumulating point of the Stomach channel.

Located 2 units superior to the lateral superior border of the patella.

Image:
The name suggests that at this point the channel Qi passes through to the lower leg by way of the area above the border or "mound" of the rectus femoris muscle. *Liang*, with the grain radical, also means "millet" and refers to this point's corresponding Organ, which is said to be like a storehouse for grain.

Functions:
Regulates the Stomach (especially Qi) and clears Heat.
> Indications: painful obstruction of the lower extremities, stomachache, gastritis, diarrhea, and acid regurgitation.

Local effect: swelling and pain of the knee and surrounding tissue.

S-35 *(dú bí)*
CALF'S NOSE

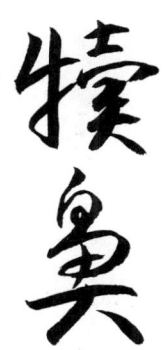

With the knee flexed, located in the depression formed by the lateral foramen of the patella.

Image:
The name refers to this point's location in a hollow next to the patellar ligament. When the knee is flexed, a hollow on each side of the knee appears, creating an impression of the nostrils of a calf. This point is also called the "eyes of the knee" when referring to both hollows.

Functions:
Benefits the knees, dispels Wind and Cold,△ and clears Heat.

    Indications: painful obstruction of the knee, pain, stiffness or inflammation of the knee and surrounding tissue, and lower leg paralysis.

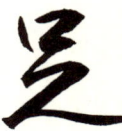

S-36 (zú sān lǐ)
FOOT THREE MILES

Sea and Earth point of the Stomach channel and Sea of Nourishment point.

Located 3 units inferior to S-35, 1 unit lateral to the anterior crest of the tibia.

Image:
The name refers to this point's strong tonifying effect, which has been used since ancient times to build up strength and endurance. It was commonly needled or moxacauterized before a person embarked upon a long journey. The number three is considered an active or Yang number. *Zu san li* can also mean "three units on the foot," which refers to its location three units below S-35 (*du bi*). *Shou san li* (LI-10), or "hand three miles," located on the arm, shares a similar relationship to its anatomical location and function.

Functions:
Regulates, strengthens and tonifies the Spleen (especially Qi and Yang), regulates the Stomach (especially Qi and Yin) and the middle and lower Burners, tonifies nutritive Qi, reduces digestive stagnation, redirects rebellious Qi downward, warms Cold,△ and drains pathogenic influences from the Stomach.

> Indications: insomnia due to stomach disorder, dysmenorrhea due to Cold, stomach and duodenal ulcers, acute and chronic gastritis, pancreatitis, childhood nutritional impairment, lack of appetite, stomachache, indigestion, diaphragmatic spasms, abdominal distention, borborygmus, and vomiting.

Regulates and tonifies the Lungs (especially Qi) and drains pathogenic influences from the Lungs.

> Indications: pulmonary tuberculosis, asthma, cough with profuse sputum, and shortness of breath.

Tonifies the Kidneys (especially Yang) and source Qi, regulates and tonifies Qi and Blood,△ facilitates Qi and Blood flow, and calms the Fetus.

> Indications: chronic consumptive disorders, chronic nephritis, restless fetus disorder due to Qi deficiency, Qi-type painful urinary dysfunction, chronic urticaria and eczema due to Blood deficiency, breast abscess, allergies, anemia, neurasthenia, late menstruation due to Blood deficiency, leukorrhea, impotence, generalized weakness, dizziness or vertigo due to Blood and Qi deficiency, headache, tinnitus, and palpitations.

Transforms Dampness and Damp-Heat, dries Dampness and Damp-Cold.△

> Indications: lower extremity atrophy syndrome, hepatitis, jaundice, acute disease of the biliary tract, and mastitis.

Regulates and moistens the Intestines.

> Indications: Intestinal Abscess, appendicitis, lower abdominal pain and distention, constipation, and diarrhea.

Alleviates exterior conditions, dispels Wind and Cold,△ clears Heat and restores collapsed Yang,△ tonifies protective Qi, and generates Fluids.

> Indications: abandoned-type Wind-stroke, Cold-predominant painful obstruction, collapsing syndrome due to deficiency, hypertension, hemiplegia, seizures, shock, facial paralysis or pain, anxiety and palpitations due to congested fluids, fatigued extremities, and acute lower back pain.

Softens hard masses.
> Indications: enlarged spleen, hard lymph nodes in the groin area, and hard abdominal masses or tumors.

Raises middle Qi.
> Indications: prolapse of various organs, particularly the stomach and intestines.

Expels stones (gallbladder and urinary tract) and parasites.
> Indications: gallbladder or kidney stones and intestinal or biliary tract parasites.

Expedites lactation.
> Indications: insufficient lactation due to deficiency.

Benefits the knees.
> Indications: various knee joint disorders including painful obstruction.

Local effect: lower leg stiffness, pain and motor impairment, and paralysis of the dorsiflexors of the foot.

S-37 *(shàng jù xū)*
UPPER GREAT VOID

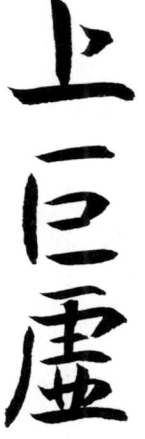

Lower Sea point of the Large Intestine channel and Sea of Blood point.

Located 6 units inferior to S-35, 1 unit lateral to the anterior crest of the tibia.

Image:
The name refers to this point's energetic function of balancing the body areas above the lower extremities, by sedating and dispersing Yang Qi excess downward and peripherally.

Functions:
Regulates the Stomach and Intestines and transforms Damp-Heat (especially Intestinal).

> Indications: acute intestinal obstruction, appendicitis, gastritis, enteritis, bacterial dysentery, abdominal pain and distention, indigestion, borborygmus, and diarrhea due to Damp-Heat.

Redirects rebellious Qi downward.

> Indications: hemiplegia, dizziness, and generalized distention.

Local effect: lower extremity stiffness and pain.

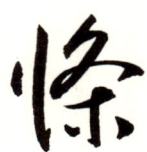
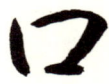

S-38 *(tiáo kǒu)*
NARROW OPENING

Located 8 units inferior to S-35, 1 unit lateral to the anterior crest of the tibia.

Image:
The name refers to this point's location in the depression of the narrow tibialis anterior muscle. *Tiao,* when combined with *feng* (wind), is also a classical term for the early spring or northeast wind and suggests this point's ability to dispel Wind.

Functions:
Regulates the Stomach.
> Indications: enteritis, stomachache, abdominal cramps, and borborygmus.

Relaxes the sinews, benefits the shoulders, and dispels Wind and Cold.[△]
> Indications: sciatica, arthritis of the knee, perifocal inflammation, shoulder pain or stiffness, frozen shoulder, dropped foot, and lower-extremity muscular cramps.

Local effect: lower leg pain, muscular atrophy and paralysis.

S-39 *(xià jù xū)*
LOWER GREAT VOID

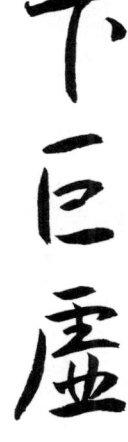

Lower Sea point of the Small Intestine channel and Sea of Blood point.

Located 9 units inferior to S-35, 1 unit lateral to the anterior crest of the tibia.

Image:
This point's function is similar to S-37 *(shang ju xu)*, except that it drains Yang Qi excess downward into the lower limbs.

Functions:
Regulates the Stomach and Intestines, transforms Damp-Heat, and redirects rebellious Qi downward.

Indications: painful obstruction of the throat, pharyngitis, acute intestinal obstruction, lower abdominal pain, back pain radiating to the testicles, diarrhea, constricted breathing, and cough.

Local effect: lower extremity pain, paralysis and muscular atrophy.

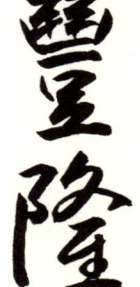

S-40 (fēng lóng)
ABUNDANT FLOURISHING

Connecting point of the Stomach channel.

Located 8 units inferior to S-35 and 2 units lateral to the anterior crest of the tibia.

Image:
The name suggests that the channel Qi is both profuse and vital here at the Connecting point. *Feng long* also means "thunder" (considered by the ancients to be a sign of earth's abundant energy) and suggests the quality of the Stomach channel Qi which, when full, overflows and is routed to the Spleen from this point.

Functions:
Regulates the Stomach and Intestines, clears Stomach Fire and Heat, drains pathogenic influences from the Lungs, transforms Dampness, Damp-Heat, Damp-Summerheat, Phlegm, Phlegm-Cold,△ Damp-Phlegm and Phlegm-Heat, and dries Dampness△ and Damp-Cold.△

> Indications: seizures, bronchitis, Lung Abscess, asthma, pertussis or pneumonia with copious sputum, Damp-predominant painful obstruction, menopausal syndrome, dizziness and vertigo due to Phlegm, vomiting, morning sickness, chest pain with difficult breathing, cough, epigastric distention and pain, loose stools or diarrhea with mucous-like discharge, difficult and painful defecation, and leg Qi.

Calms the Spirit and transforms Heart Phlegm.

> Indications: depression and mania due to Phlegm, incoherent speech, chest pain and palpitations with anxiety and insomnia.

Dispels Wind and Wind-Phlegm.

Indications: painful obstruction of the throat and fatigued extremities, intercostal neuralgia, facial paralysis with copious sputum, lower limb paralysis due to stroke, dizziness, and headache.

Local effect: lower limb pain, paralysis, swelling or muscular atrophy.

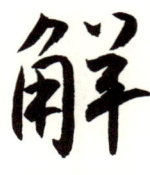

S-41 (jiě xī)
RELEASE STREAM

River and Fire point of the Stomach channel.

Located level with the vertex of the lateral malleolus on the anterior aspect of the ankle joint between the tendons of the extensor digitorum longus and hallucis longus muscles.

Image:
The name suggests that this point releases or unblocks stagnant channel Qi flow and releases ankle joint restriction. *Jie*, which denotes separation, refers to this point's location in the depression formed by the ankle joint; its classical meaning, "untie," refers to the place on the foot where the shoes were tied.

Functions:
Regulates the Stomach (especially Qi), clears Stomach Fire and Heat, and dispels Wind.
> Indications: seizures, lower extremity atrophy syndrome, delirium due to Stomach Fire, head and facial edema, eye redness, headache, dizziness, vomiting due to Stomach Heat, abdominal distention, and constipation.

Calms the Spirit and clears the Brain.
> Indications: mania, depression, incoherent speech, and chest pain.

Local effect: lower leg pain, stiffness or muscular atrophy.

S-42 (chōng yáng)
RUSHING YANG

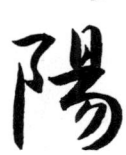

Source point of the Stomach channel.

Located 1.3 units distal to S-41 at the highest point of the dorsum of the foot in the depression formed by the second and third metatarsal bones and the cuneiform bone.

Image:

The name suggests the active, intense and vital nature of the channel Qi flow at this point. *Chong* may also allude to the Penetrating vessel which crosses this point (see *Spiritual Axis*, chapter 38).

Functions:

Regulates the Stomach.
> Indications: lack of appetite, epigastric pain and distention, abdominal distention, and constipation.

Calms the Spirit.
> Indications: hysteria, anxiety, and chronic restlessness.

Clears Stomach Fire and Heat and dispels Wind.
> Indications: malarial disorders, fever, facial paralysis with swelling, facial edema, gingivitis, toothache, and leg Qi.

Local effect: muscular atrophy, weakness and pain of the foot and swelling of the dorsum of the foot.

S-43 *(xiàn gǔ)*
DEEP VALLEY

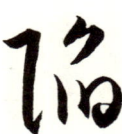

Stream and Wood point of the Stomach channel.

Located in the depression distal to the junction of the second and third metatarsal bones.

Image:
The name refers to this point's location on the Stomach channel where it passes through a deep "valley" between the second and third metatarsal bones.

Functions:
Regulates the Stomach and transforms Dampness.
> Indications: facial or general edema, epigastric or abdominal pain, and borborygmus.

Dispels Wind and clears Heat.
> Indications: seizures, tonsillitis, conjunctivitis, and generalized muscular aches.

Local effect: pain and swelling of dorsum of foot, dropped foot or heel pain.

S-44 (nèi tíng)
INNER COURTYARD

Spring and Water point of the Stomach channel.

Located proximal to the web margin between the second and third toes in the depression distal and lateral to the second metatarsal phalangeal joint.

Image:
The name refers to this point's location in the interdigital area between the second and third toes.

Functions:
Regulates the Stomach (especially Qi) and Intestines, transforms Damp-Heat, and drains pathogenic influences from the Stomach.

> Indications: dysenteric disorders or diarrhea due to Damp-Heat, acute or chronic enteritis, constipation due to Heat, epigastric pain or hiccups, abdominal pain and distention, and morning sickness.

Dispels Wind-Heat, reduces fever, clears Stomach Fire and Heat, regulates Qi, and alleviates pain.

> Indications: febrile diseases, urticaria, trigeminal neuralgia, facial paralysis, lockjaw, pain due to intestinal hernia, poor appetite, stomachache, diaphragmatic spasms, fever without sweating, toothache, frontal headache, epistaxis, sore throat, and dysmenorrhea.

Local effect: pain and swelling of the dorsum of the foot.

S-45 (lì duì)
EVIL'S DISSIPATION

Well and Metal point of the Stomach channel.

Located about 0.1 unit from the lateral corner of the second toenail.

Image:
The name suggests this point's ability to uplift and calm the Spirit by dispelling external forces. *Li*, when combined with *feng*, suggests a violent wind; with *gui* it suggests an evil spirit. In ancient times, being attacked by wind implied being possessed or disturbed by a spirit. When combined with the classical meaning for *dui* (pronounced *yue*), which means "to use words that dispel grief and please the ear," the image is completed.

Functions:
Regulates the Stomach, clears Heat, and transforms Damp-Heat.
> Indications: hepatitis, abdominal Heat, abdominal or epigastric pain, indigestion, facial edema, tonsillitis, sore throat, toothache, epistaxis, and yellow nasal discharge.

Calms the Spirit.
> Indications: hysteria, depression, disorientation, and dream-disturbed sleep.

Local effect: cold and numbness of the toes and feet.

Sp-1 (yǐn bái)
HIDDEN CLARITY

Well and Wood point of the Spleen channel.

Located about 0.1 unit from the medial corner of the first toenail.

Image:
The name suggests this point's capacity to instill clarity of thought and mind, which correlates to the Spleen's Spirit aspect of intelligence, or *yi* (see B-49 *[yi she]*). *Yin bai* can also mean "hidden white," referring to the area of white flesh where the point is located.

Functions:
Regulates and tonifies the Spleen (especially Yang) and facilitates Blood flow.

> Indications: childhood convulsions, lack of appetite, prolonged menstruation, nausea, abdominal distention, chest and epigastric fullness and pain, and sudden diarrhea.

Contains the Blood.$^\triangle$

> Indications: all types of bleeding due to Spleen deficiency including epistaxis, abnormal uterine bleeding, and blood in the urine or stool.

Calms the Spirit and clears the Brain.

> Indications: mania, depression, melancholia, convulsions, insomnia, and dream-disturbed sleep.

Sp-2 (dà dū)
GREAT CAPITAL

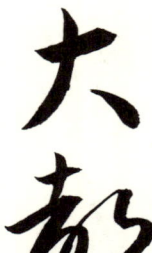

Spring and Fire point of the Spleen channel.

Located on the medial side of the first toe distal and inferior to the first metatarsophalangeal joint at the junction of the red and white skin.

Image:
The name refers to a gathering place for Qi within the channel, giving the point great influence, like the capital of a country.

Functions:
Regulates the Spleen (especially Qi and Yang) and Stomach (especially Qi) and reduces digestive stagnation.

> Indications: restlessness with insomnia, sensation of heaviness of the body with swelling at the extremities, sensation of fullness and tightness in the chest, vomiting, epigastric pain, abdominal distention, poor digestion, belching, borborygmus, diarrhea, and constipation.

Sp-3 (tài bái)
GREAT BRIGHTNESS

Source, Stream and Earth point of the Spleen channel.

Located proximal and inferior to the head of the first metatarsal bone at the junction of the red and white skin.

Image:
This is the name for the planet Venus, which corresponds to metal of the five phases. To ancient astrologers, Venus signified the warrior (the planet's movement in the sky was believed to correspond to military conflicts on earth) who put down uprisings and regained peace. Similarly, this point affects initial stage-acute conditions of the Large Intestine, the Yang metal Organ.

Functions:
Regulates and strengthens the Spleen (especially Qi and Yang), regulates the Stomach (especially Qi and Yin) and Large Intestine, middle and lower Burners, clears Heat, reduces digestive stagnation, and transforms Dampness and Damp-Heat.

> Indications: dysenteric disorders, acute gastroenteritis, hunger with no desire to eat, sensation of heaviness of the body with arthritic pain, edema, nausea, vomiting, hypochondriac, abdominal or stomach pain and distention, headache, borborygmus, belching, indigestion, constipation, and diarrhea.

Sp-4 (gōng sūn)

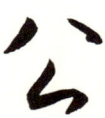
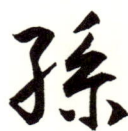

ANCESTOR AND DESCENDANT

Connecting point of the Spleen channel, Confluent point of the Penetrating vessel.

Located approximately 1 unit posterior to Sp-3 in the depression distal and inferior to the base of the first metatarsal bone at the junction of the red and white skin.

Image:
The name refers to this point's role as a Confluent point of the Penetrating vessel and a Connecting point linking the Spleen and Stomach channels. The Penetrating vessel is closely associated with source Qi that is passed on to the fetus by the parents at conception. The Spleen and Stomach are the Organs responsible for nutrition. *Sun* is also the name for the Lesser Connecting channels and *gong* also means "common" or "collective," suggesting this point's classification as a Connecting point. The Yellow Emperor, surnamed *Gong-Sun*, has been credited with discovering this point.

Functions:
Regulates and strengthens the Spleen (especially Qi and Yang), regulates the Stomach (especially Qi), middle and lower Burners, reduces digestive stagnation, tonifies source Qi, clears Heat, transforms Dampness and Damp-Heat (especially Spleen and Stomach), and invigorates the Blood.

> Indications: dysenteric disorders, stomach or upper abdominal pain due to Blood stasis, suppressed appetite in pulmonary tuberculosis, acute and chronic enteritis, jaundice, tidal fever, edema, vomiting, upper digestive-tract bleeding, intestinal clumping,

indigestion, abdominal distention, leg Qi, and chronic loose stools or diarrhea.

Calms the Spirit and clears the Brain.

Indications: seizures, mania with incoherent speech, hysteria with hiccups, excessive sleepiness, and restlessness.

Regulates the Penetrating vessel and menstruation.

Indications: endometriosis, irregular or late menstruation, morning sickness, chest pain, and lower abdominal pain.

Sp-5 (shāng qiū)
METAL'S NOTE HILL

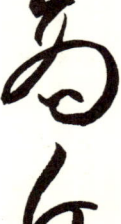

River and Metal point of the Spleen channel.

Located in the depression distal and inferior to the medial malleolus halfway between the tuberosity of the navicular bone and the vertex of the medial malleolus.

Image:
Hill refers to this point's location on the upper dorsal aspect of the foot. *Metal's note* refers to this point's classification as a Metal point and the musical note which corresponds to the metal phase.

Functions:
Regulates and strengthens the Spleen, regulates the Stomach and middle Burner, and transforms Damp-Heat.

> Indications: jaundice, gastritis, enteritis, lassitude, excessive appetite, poor digestion, abdominal distention, stomachache, flatulence, diarrhea, and constipation.

Local effect: pain and stiffness of the ankle and foot, pain along the inner part of the leg and knee.

Sp-6 *(sān yīn jiāo)*
THREE YIN JUNCTION

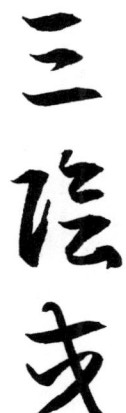

Intersecting point of the Liver and Kidney channels on the Spleen channel.

Located 3 units directly superior to the vertex of the medial malleolus on the posterior border of the tibia.

Image:
The name refers to this point's intersection with the three Yin channels of the foot.

Functions:
Regulates, strengthens and tonifies the Spleen (especially Qi and Yang), regulates the Stomach (especially Qi), middle and lower Burners, reduces digestive stagnation, tonifies Qi△ and Blood,△ nourishes Blood Dryness, facilitates Blood flow, clears Fire due to deficiency.

> Indications: hyperthyroidism, pancreatitis, enteritis, insomnia, edema, spontaneous or night sweating, dizziness and vertigo due to Qi and Blood deficiency, fatigued extremities, leg Qi, lower abdominal fullness and distention, flatulence, and chronic loose stools or diarrhea with abdominal pain.

Resolves Dampness and Damp-Heat (especially Spleen and Stomach) and dries Dampness△ and Damp-Cold.△

> Indications: dysenteric disorders due to Damp-Cold, hepatitis, eczema, urticaria, urinary tract infection due to Damp-Heat, cloudy urine, and leukorrhea.

Tonifies the Kidneys (especially Yin) and Essence, stabilizes Kidney Qi and lower orifices, enriches Yin, regulates the Water Pathways, promotes urination, and moistens Dryness.

Indications: hypertension due to Kidney Yin deficiency, painful urinary dysfunction, nephritis, prostatitis, impotence, sterility, neurasthenia, renal colic, urinary tract infection, urinary incontinence or retention, spermatorrhea or irregular menstruation due to pulmonary tuberculosis, insomnia, emaciation and weakness, and lower back and knee pain.

Regulates menstruation, warms Cold,$^\triangle$ invigorates the Blood, cools Heat in the Blood, expedites labor, and calms the Fetus.

Indications: all types of bleeding including abnormal uterine bleeding, aborted dead fetus, restless fetus disorder due to deficiency, stomachache due to Blood stasis, menopausal syndrome, amenorrhea, dysmenorrhea, morning sickness, difficult labor, and retained placenta.

Regulates the Liver (especially Yin), subdues Liver Yang, and regulates Qi.

Indications: hysteria with sudden laughing and crying, testicular mumps, irregular menstruation, generalized weakness, and dizziness.

Raises middle Qi.

Indications: organ prolapse of the abdominal region including hernial disorders and uterine prolapse.

Softens hard masses.

Indications: enlarged spleen, cirrhosis of the liver, scrofula, inguinal lymphandenitis, and hard abdominal masses or tumors.

Local effect: lower extremity pain, muscular atrophy, paralysis and motor impairment and pain on the medial side of the ankle.

Needling contraindicated during pregnancy.

Sp-8 (dì jī)
EARTH'S MECHANISM

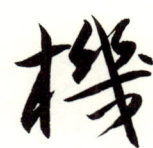

Accumulating point of the Spleen channel.

Located 3 units inferior to the medial condyle of the tibia on the line connecting Sp-9 and the medial malleolus.

Image:
The name refers to this point's main function as the controlling mechanism for regulation of the Spleen, and to its location on the lower portion of the body below the umbilicus, both of which correspond to the earth phase.

Functions:
Regulates and tonifies the Spleen (especially Qi), regulates and tonifies the Blood, invigorates the Blood, and regulates menstruation.

> Indications: amenorrhea due to Blood stasis, dysmenorrhea, irregular menstruation, abnormal uterine bleeding, edema, abdominal and flank distention, lower back pain, difficult urination, leukorrhea, and diarrhea.

Stabilizes Kidney Qi.

> Indications: infertility, spermatorrhea, urinary incontinence, chills, stiffness and pain of the lower back and knee.

Sp-9 (yīn líng quán)
YIN MOUND SPRING

Sea and Water point of the Spleen channel.

Located on the inferior border of the medial condyle of the tibia in a depression between the posterior border of the tibia and the gastrocnemius muscle.

Image:
This point is located in a depression or opening at the inferior margin of the epicondyle of the tibia, like a spring at the base of a hill or mound. *Yin spring* refers to a deep and pure source of Yin energy.

Functions:
Regulates and tonifies the Spleen (especially Yang), regulates the Stomach (especially Yin) and lower Burner, resolves Dampness and Damp-Heat (especially Spleen-Stomach) and Damp-Summerheat, regulates the Water Pathways, and promotes urination.

> Indications: atrophy syndrome due to Damp-Heat, Damp-Heat painful obstruction, hypertension due to Dampness, painful urinary obstruction, diarrhea with undigested food or mucus due to Damp-Heat, hepatitis, jaundice, acute nephritis, ascites, edema, urticaria, stomachache, lack of appetite, abdominal distention, lower abdominal cold and pain, lower back pain, urinary tract infection, urinary retention or incontinence, and leukorrhea.

Sp-10 (xuè hǎi)
SEA OF BLOOD

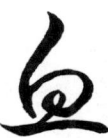
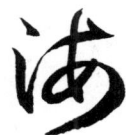

With the knee flexed, located 2 units superior to the medial superior ridge of the patella.

Image:
The name refers to this point's major role in the regulation and distribution of Blood.

Functions:
Regulates the Spleen (especially Qi) and menstruation, calms the Fetus, regulates and tonifies the Blood,△ invigorates the Blood, facilitates Blood flow, tonifies nutritive Qi, clears Heat and Summerheat, cools Heat in the Blood and nourishes Blood Dryness.

> Indications: all types of bleeding including Blood-type painful urinary dysfunction, restless fetus disorder due to Heat in the Blood or Blood deficiency, early menstruation due to Heat in the Blood, eczema and urticaria due to Heat in the Blood, abnormal uterine bleeding due to Heat in the Blood, amenorrhea, irregular menstruation, dysmenorrhea, testicular mumps, malarial disorders, herpes zoster, vaginal pruritis, anemia, generalized itching, and abdominal fullness.

Local effect: pain in medial thigh area.

Sp-12 (chōng mén)
PENETRATING GATE

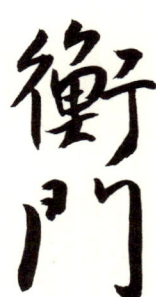

Intersecting point of the Liver channel on the Spleen channel.

Located 3.5 units lateral to CV-2 on the lateral side of the femoral artery at the level of the upper border of the pubic symphysis.

Image:
The name suggests a passageway into the interior. This point is situated in an area known as the "Qi corridor" at the border of the trunk and leg, where the Qi tends to stagnate, and suggests this point's role in maintaining proper Qi flow through the corridor. (Some merely associate the Qi corridor with the femoral artery.) *Chong* also refers to the Penetrating vessel which has a branch that descends through this region, suggesting this point's area of influence.

Functions:
Transforms Damp-Heat, facilitates Qi and Blood flow.

Indications: hernial disorders, painful urinary dysfunction, gestational edema, abdominal pain and distention, urinary retention, orchitis, endometriosis, and leukorrhea.

CAUTION: *avoid puncturing artery.*

Sp-15 *(dà héng)*
GREAT TRANSVERSE

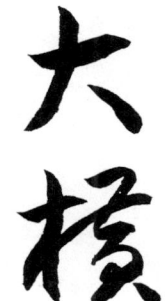

Intersecting point of the Yin-linking vessel on the Spleen channel.

Located 4 units lateral to the center of the umbilicus on the midclavicular line.

Image:
The name refers to this point's location at the intersection of the transverse line through the umbilicus and the vertical line through the nipple. In addition, the name and location of this point (directly above the Large Intestine, or *da chang*) suggests a relationship between the point and its neighboring Organ.

Functions:
Regulates the Spleen (especially Qi), regulates and moistens the Intestines, reduces digestive stagnation and transforms Damp-Heat (especially intestinal).

> Indications: dysenteric disorders with or without Blood, appendicitis, abdominal distention, lower abdominal pain or cold, fatigued extremities, constipation, severe diarrhea, and fecal incontinence.

Expels parasites (intestinal).

Sp-21 (dà bāo)
GREAT ENVELOPE

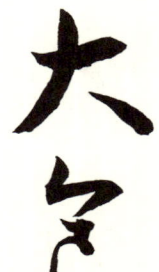

Special Connecting point of the Spleen channel.

Located in the sixth intercostal space on the mid-axillary line midway between the axilla (H-1) and the free end of the eleventh rib (Liv-13).

Image:
From this point Blood and nutritive Qi are distributed and regulated. These substances "envelop" the body. The original character for *bao* meant "a fetus in a womb," which supports the image of nurturing and enveloping.

Functions:
Expands and relaxes the chest, regulates Qi and Blood, tonifies nutritive Qi, facilitates Qi and Blood flow.

> Indications: generalized body pain and aches, lethargy and depression, intercostal neuralgia, chest and hypochondriac fullness and pain, asthma, cough, dyspnea, emaciation due to prolonged illness, and fatigued extremities.

H-1 *(jí quán)*
UTMOST SPRING

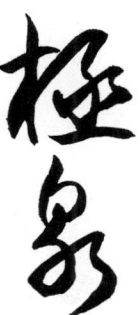

Located at the center of the axilla on the medial side of the axillary artery.

Image:
The name suggests that from this point channel Qi flows down from the "spring" at the channel's external origin in the axilla toward the hands below. The name also evokes the idea of the Qi at its zenith, when it is most intense and abundant.

Functions:
Regulates the Heart, expands and relaxes the chest, facilitates Qi flow.

    Indications: jaundice, intercostal neuralgia, oppressive sensation in the hypochondrium, chest pain, nausea, poor vision, and excessive thirst.

Local effect: pain, cold and the inability to raise the arm.

H-2 (qīng líng)
GREEN SPIRIT

With elbow flexed, located 3 units above H-3 in the groove medial to the biceps brachii muscle.

Image:
The name suggests corporeal and spiritual renewal. *Qing* refers to the natural hue of plants; *ling* refers to offerings made to the deities for rain to replenish the earth. Together they suggest spiritual regeneration (the Heart stores the Spirit and is the root of life).

Functions:
Expands and relaxes the chest, regulates Qi and Blood and clears Heat.

> Indications: body tremors, chest or epigastric pain, intercostal pain or neuralgia, inability to raise the arm, shoulder and arm stiffness, inflammation, pain or paralysis, headache, jaundiced eyes, and fever.

H-3 *(shào hǎi)*
LESSER SEA

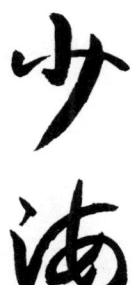

Sea and Water point of the Heart channel.

With the elbow flexed, located at the medial end of the transverse cubital crease in the depression anterior to the medial epicondyle of the humerus.

Image:
Sea refers to this point's classification as a Sea point where the channel Qi gathers together. *Lesser* suggests its location on the Hand Lesser Yin channel.

Functions:
Regulates the Heart (especially Qi) and regulates Qi and Blood.
> Indications: chest pain with nausea and vomiting, axilla and hypochondriac pain, arm numbness, hand tremors, intercostal neuralgia, fever and chills, sudden loss of voice, headache, and dizziness.

Calms the Spirit and strengthens the Brain.
> Indications: seizures, neurasthenia, forgetfulness, and disorientation.

Local effect: contracture and pain of the elbow.

H-4 (líng dào)
SPIRIT'S PATH

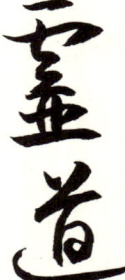

River and Metal point of the Heart channel.

With the palm facing upward, located 1.5 units above the transverse crease of the wrist on the radial side of the tendon of the flexor carpi ulnaris muscle.

Image:
The name refers to this point's effect on the Spirit (which is governed by the Heart) and suggests a pathway for the Spirit's energies to travel along.

Functions:
Regulates the Heart.
> Indications: sensation of cold in the bones, aphasia with stiffening of the tongue, convulsions, chest pain, palpitations, retching, nausea, eye redness, sudden loss of voice, dizziness, and blurred vision.

Calms the Spirit.
> Indications: hysteria, restlessness, fear and melancholia, incoherent thinking or speech.

Local effect: contracture of the elbow and arm.

H-5 (tōng lǐ)
COMMUNICATION'S ROUTE

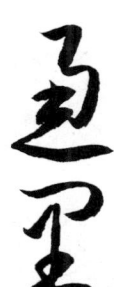

Connecting point of the Heart channel.
Located 1 unit proximal to H-7, on a line connecting H-7 and H-4.

Image:
This is the Connecting point of the Heart channel, which communicates with the Small Intestine channel. *Tong* refers to quick and clear thinking and communication, also suggesting this point's function in enhancing mental acuity.

Functions:
Regulates and tonifies the Heart (especially the Qi and Yang).
> Indications: Wind-stroke with aphasia and stiffening of the tongue, sensation of heaviness of the body, fatigue, dizziness, blurred vision, chest pain, palpitations due to fright, arrhythmia, sudden voice loss or hoarseness of the voice, and headache.

Clears Heart Fire and deficiency Heat.
> Indications: hypertension due to Heart Fire excess, fever with chest discomfort, sweating, menorrhagia, abnormal uterine bleeding, and urinary incontinence.

Calms the Spirit and strengthens the Brain.
> Indications: insanity, depression or hysteria with aphasia, neurasthenia, somnolence or insomnia, palpitations due to fright, and fear of people.

Local effect: pain in the wrist and arm.

H-6 (yīn xì)
YIN'S CREVICE

Accumulating point of the Heart channel.

Located 0.5 unit proximal to H-7 on a line connecting H-7 to H-4.

Image:
The name refers to this point's location on a Yin channel between two tendons of the wrist muscles, which form a crevice or narrow opening where the Qi and Blood collect. *Xi* is the term for an Accumulating point.

Functions:
Regulates and tonifies the Heart (especially Yin and Blood), enriches Yin, transforms Heart Phlegm, invigorates the Blood, and facilitates Blood flow.

> Indications: stiffness and pain along the Heart channel due to stagnant Heart Blood, stifling sensation or pain in the chest, sudden chest pain, sudden loss of voice, palpitations, and aphasia.

Clears deficiency Heat and cools Heat in the Blood.

> Indications: pulmonary tuberculosis with night sweats due to Yin deficiency, spontaneous sweating or night sweats, hemoptysis, and epistaxis.

Calms the Spirit and clears the Brain.

> Indications: hysteria, fright, grief, sudden irritability and rage, anxiety and palpitations.

H-7 (shén mén)
SPIRIT'S GATE

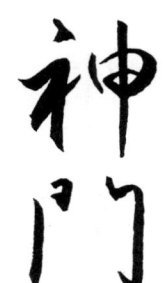

Source, Stream and Earth point of the Heart channel.

Located on the transverse wrist crease on the radial side of the tendon of the flexor carpi ulnaris muscle.

Image:
The name refers to a "gateway" on the Heart channel through which the Organ's host energy (the Spirit) is directly affected. In Taoism, *shen men* refers to the eyes (which reflect the presence and strength of the Spirit), the place where the Spirit enters and exits.

Functions:
Regulates and tonifies the Heart (especially Qi, Blood, Yin and Yang), transforms Heart Phlegm, and benefits the tongue.

> Indications: sensation of the heart being enlarged, chest pain with palpitations, arrhythmia, dizziness, headache, paralysis of the hyoglossus muscle of the tongue, aphasia, asthmatic wheezing, malaise, and neurasthenia.

Clears Heart Fire, Heat, deficiency Heat and cools Heat in the Blood.

> Indications: Hypertension, hyperthyroidism with dream-disturbed sleep, feverish sensation in the palms due to deficiency, desire for cold drinks, fever and chills (chills predominant), lack of appetite with painful obstruction of the throat, hemoptysis, bloody stool, and eczema with intense itching.

Calms the Spirit, strengthens and clears the Brain, and dispels Wind-Phlegm.

Indications: insanity, mania, seizures, mental retardation, pulmonary tuberculosis with irritability and insomnia, depression, hyperactivity, restlessness, fright, anxiety and palpitations, insomnia, dream-disturbed sleep, delirious speech, forgetfulness, disorientation, urinary incontinence, impotence, and nocturnal emission.

H-8 (shào fǔ)
LESSER PALACE

Spring and Fire point of the Heart channel.

Located on the transverse crease of the palm halfway between the fourth and fifth metacarpal bones.

Image:
The name suggests a wayside palace where a monarch rests. (*Simple Questions* refers to the Heart as the "monarch" of the body.) *Shao fu* is also a classical term for the official whose rank placed him in charge of storage, suggesting this point's ability to harbor the Spirit. In addition, *fu* (with the flesh radical) is a term for the Yang Organs, suggesting this point's effect on the Heart's related Organ, the Small Intestine.

Functions:
Regulates the Heart (especially Qi), benefits the tongue, and transforms Heart Phlegm.

> Indications: palpitations, arrhythmia, chest fullness and pain, somnolence, fatigue, tongue contracture and stiffness.

Clears Heart Fire and Heat, Heat (especially Small Intestine), transforms Damp-Heat (especially lower Burner), and drains pathogenic influences from the Heart.

> Indications: vaginal pain or pruritis, uterine prolapse, dysuria, urinary retention, urinary incontinence, carbuncles and boils, and sensation of heat in the palms.

Calms the Spirit.

> Indications: mania with frequent laughing, grief, fear, and fright.

Local effect: twisting and contracture of the small finger.

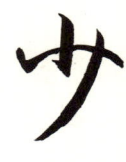
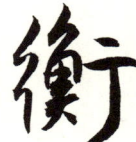

H-9 *(shào chōng)*
LESSER RUSHING

Well and Wood point of the Heart channel.

Located about 0.1 unit from the radial corner of the fifth fingernail.

Image:
This point is situated at the end of the Heart channel, where the channel Qi quickly rushes into the interior. *Lesser* denotes the quantity of Qi or the location of this point on the Hand Lesser Yin channel.

Functions:
Regulates the Heart.
> Indications: chest pain, arrhythmia, palpitations, and numbness in the arm and small finger.

Clears Heart Fire, cools Heat in the Blood, and redirects rebellious Qi downward.
> Indications: febrile diseases, jaundice, sore throat, hemoptysis, and bloody stool with mucus.

Revives consciousness and clears the Brain.
> Indications: coma due to Wind-stroke, mania, severe depression, and sudden loss of consciousness.

Local effect: pain along the posterior medial aspect of the upper limbs.

SI-1 *(shào zé)*
YOUNG MARSH

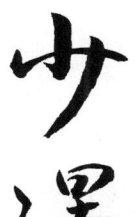

Well and Metal point of the Small Intestine channel.

Located about 0.1 unit from the ulnar corner of the fifth fingernail.

Image:
The name refers to this point's location, where the channel Qi gathers like a marsh to form the first point of the external channel's course. The name also reflects the point's function of moistening Dryness and clearing Heat.

Functions:
Dispels Wind-Heat, clears Heat, and moistens Dryness.

> Indications: convulsions due to Heat, fever and chills, headache, epistaxis, sore throat, dry mouth, neck pain, chest and intercostal pain, and shortness of breath.

Revives consciousness and opens the sensory orifices.

> Indications: Wind-stroke, collapsing syndrome, deafness, tinnitus, and tongue stiffness.

Expedites and facilitates lactation.

> Indications: mastitis and insufficient lactation.

Local effect: pain along the posterior-lateral aspect of the upper extremity.

SI-2 (qián gŭ)
FORWARD VALLEY

Spring and Water point of the Small Intestine channel.

With a loose fist, located distal to the metacarpophalangeal joint in the depression at the junction of the red and white skin.

Image:
The name refers to this point's location and describes the channel Qi as it moves from SI-1 (*shao ze*) into a valley or depression.

Functions:
Dispels Wind-Heat.
> Indications: seizures, high fever without sweating, nasal obstruction, and pain and stiffness of the neck and back.

Opens the ears.
> Indications: deafness, tinnitus, and swollen jaw with pain radiating to the back of the ear.

Moistens the throat.
> Indications: mumps, throat pain, soreness and dryness, and cough.

Local effect: pain and inflammation of the finger joints, finger numbness and contracture of the elbow.

SI-3 (hòu xī)
BACK STREAM

Stream and Wood point of the Small Intestine channel and Confluent point of the Governing vessel.

With a loose fist, located proximal to the head of the fifth metacarpal bone on the ulnar side in the depression at the junction of the red and white skin.

Image:

The name refers to the intense and vital nature of the channel Qi flow at this point, which resembles a *stream*, and its position in back of the metacarpophalangeal joint. *Back* may also refer to this point's influence on the Governing vessel.

Functions:

Releases exterior conditions, stimulates sweating, dispels Wind and Wind-Heat, clears Fire, Heat and Summerheat, and drains pathogenic influences from the Heart.

> Indications: febrile diseases without sweating, malarial disorders, scabies, common cold with fever and red eyes, tidal fever, dizziness and vertigo, dry mouth, conjunctivitis, and epistaxis.

Regulates the Governing vessel, relaxes the sinews, benefits the joints, and alleviates pain.

> Indications: Painful obstruction with generalized aches, muscular tetany, occipital or parietal headache, neck or upper back stiffness and pain, whiplash, spinal pain or stiffness, and contracture and twitching of the arm, elbow and fingers.

Calms the Spirit, clears the Brain, transforms Heart Phlegm, and dispels Wind-Phlegm.

Indications: collapsing syndrome due to excess Heat, convulsions, hysteria, mania, seizures, melancholia, insomnia, dream-disturbed sleep with night sweating, and deaf-mutism.

Local effect: hand and finger pain and motor impairment.

SI-4 (wàn gǔ)
WRIST BONE

Source point of the Small Intestine channel.

Located on the ulnar side of the palm in the depression between the fifth metacarpal bone and the hamate and pisiform bones.

Image:
The name is a classical term for the carpal bones and refers to this point's location and area of influence.

Functions:
Relaxes the sinews, dispels Wind-Heat, clears Heat, and transforms Damp-Heat.

> Indications: malarial disorders, painful obstruction of the throat, pediatric convulsions, jaundice, fever, mumps, upper extremity arthritis, neck stiffness or inflammation, pain in the hypochondrium, and gastritis.

Local effect: all wrist problems including pain, inflammation, contracture and wrist and finger stiffness.

SI-5 (yáng gǔ)
YANG VALLEY

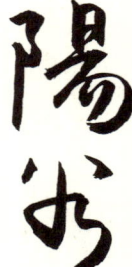

River and Fire point of the Small Intestine channel.

Located on the ulnar side of the wrist in a depression between the styloid process of the ulna and the triquetral bone.

Image:
The name is an anatomical reference: *valley* refers to the depression between the styloid process of the ulna and the triquetral bone where this point is located; *yang* refers to this point's location on the Yang region of the hand.

Functions:
Clears Heat and dispels Wind-Heat.
> Indications: scabies, fever without sweating, dizziness, swelling of the neck and submandibular region, mumps and toothache.

Opens the sensory orifices, calms the Spirit, and clears the Brain.
> Indications: mania, convulsions, fright, delirium, depression, incoherent speech, tongue stiffness, deafness, tinnitus, and eye redness and pain.

Local effect: pain in the wrist and lateral aspect of the arm.

SI-6 (yǎng lǎo)
SUPPORTING THE OLD

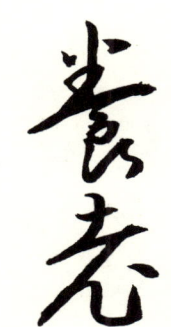

Accumulating point of the Small Intestine channel.

With the palm facing the chest, located in the bony cleft on the radial side of the styloid process of the ulna.

Image:
The name refers to this point's ability to revitalize the Qi in the joints and sinews where Qi obstruction commonly occurs in the elderly.

Functions:
Relaxes the sinews and benefits the joints.
> Indications: hemiplegia, neck stiffness, arthritis of the upper extremities, acute lower back pain or restriction of movement, shoulder and back pain, and shoulder, elbow and arm pain.

Brightens the eyes.
> Indications: blurred vision, dull eye pain, and sunken and heavy feeling of the eye.

Local effect: pain in the elbow and forearm.

SI-7 (zhī zhèng)
BRANCH FROM THE MAIN

Connecting point of the Small Intestine channel.

Located 5 units proximal to the wrist on the line connecting SI-5 and SI-8.

Image:
This is the exit point from the main channel to the Connecting channel or branch.

Functions:
Dispels Wind, clears Heat and stimulates sweating.
> Indications: febrile diseases without sweating, headache, vertigo, neck stiffness, pain, paralysis or weakness of the shoulder and neck, and fatigued extremities.

Calms the Spirit and clears the Brain.
> Indications: hysteria, mania, neurasthenia, fright, and anxiety.

Local effect: pain in the elbow and forearm.

SI-8 *(xiǎo hǎi)*
SMALL SEA

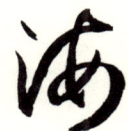

Sea and Earth point of the Small Intestine channel.

With the elbow flexed, located halfway between the olecranon of the ulna and medial epicondyle of the humerus.

Image:
The name refers to the gathering of channel Qi at this point and its classification as a Sea point.

Functions:
Dispels Wind and relaxes the sinews.
> Indications: seizures, convulsions, fever with chills, dizziness and vertigo, headache, neck and shoulder stiffness, inflammation and pain.

Local effect: pain and stiffness of the elbow and arm.

SI-9 *(jiān zhēn)*
SHOULDER INTEGRITY

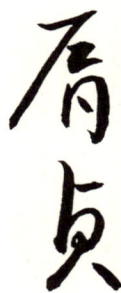

With the arm abducted, located 1 unit superior to the posterior end of the axillary fold.

Image:
The name refers to this point's role in maintaining proper shoulder joint function.

Functions:
Benefits the shoulders and dispels Wind.
> Indications: pain, stiffness, paralysis or arthritis of the scapula, shoulder and arm, neck pain and inflammation, arm weakness and soreness, excessive underarm perspiration, and tinnitus.

SI-10 (nào shū)
SCAPULA'S HOLLOW

Intersecting point of the Yang-linking and Yang-heel vessels on the Small Intestine channel.

With the arm abducted, located directly superior to SI-9 in the depression inferior and lateral to the scapular spine.

Image:
The name refers to this point's direct effect upon the scapula. *Hollow* suggests a container or conveyor through which the circulating Qi passes (see B-13 *[fei shu]*).

Functions:
Dispels Wind and benefits the shoulders.

> Indications: pain, stiffness, paralysis or arthritis of the scapula, shoulder and arm, soreness and lack of strength in the arm, and neck pain and inflammation.

Softens hard masses.

> Indications: lymphadenitis, scrofula.

SI-11 *(tiān zōng)*
HEAVEN'S WORSHIP

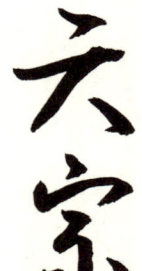

Located 1 unit inferior to the midpoint of the lower border of the scapular spine.

Image:
The name, a general term for a celestial phenomenon, refers to the "constellation" of points positioned relatively equadistant around this point (those on the adjacent Small Intestine and Bladder channels), and to this point's influence on them.

Functions:
Expands and relaxes the chest, dispels Wind, redirects rebellious Qi downward.

> Indications: asthma, cough, severe and painful hiccups, pain in the shoulder and shoulder blade, cheek and jaw swelling.

Facilitates lactation.

> Indications: mastitis.

SI-12 *(bǐng fēng)*
HOLDS WIND

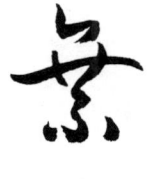
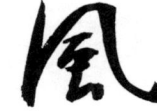

Intersecting point of the Gallbladder, Triple Burner and Large Intestine channels on the Small Intestine channel.

Located 1 unit superior to the midpoint of the upper border of the scapular spine.

Image:
The name suggests this point's vulnerability to externally-contracted Wind.

Functions:
Benefits the shoulders, dispels Wind and Cold,△ and clears Heat.

    Indications: all shoulder and scapular problems, shoulder and arm neuralgia and numbness.

SI-15 *(jiān zhōng shū)*
MIDDLE SHOULDER HOLLOW

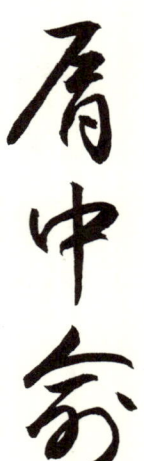

Located 2 units lateral to the lower border of the spinous process of the seventh cervical vertebra (GV-14).

Image:
The name refers to this point's specific effect on the shoulder and the upper chest and its location on the back of the shoulder near the Governing channel at the midpoint of the line connecting GV-14 and GB-21. The word *hollow* suggests a container or conveyor through which the circulating Qi passes (see B-13 *[fei shu]*).

Functions:
Diffuses Lung Qi, clears Heat, benefits the shoulders, and transforms Phlegm and Phlegm-Heat.

Indications: bronchitis, asthma, bronchiectasis, shortness of breath, cough, fever and chills, sensation of heat and cold in the back, various shoulder disorders, spitting up of blood, and dypsnea.

Local effect: pain, inflammation and stiffness of the shoulder, neck and upper back.

SI-17 *(tiān róng)*
HEAVEN'S RECEPTION

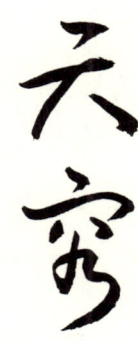

Posterior to and level with the angle of the mandible, located in the depression on the anterior border of the sternocleidomastoid muscle.

Image:
The name refers to the place where the channel Qi is received by and enters into the "heaven body zone" (the head or skull).

Functions:
Moistens the throat, and clears Heat.
> Indications: painful obstruction of the throat with difficulty swallowing, neck swelling and soreness, tonsillitis, pharyngitis, and tinnitus.

Softens hard masses.
> Indications: neck lumps or abscesses, scrofula, and goiter.

SI-18 (quán liáo)
CHEEKBONE OPENING

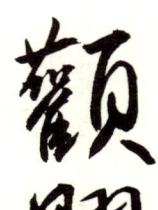

Intersecting point of the Triple Burner channel on the Small Intestine channel.

Located on the lower border of the zygomatic bone directly below the outer canthus.

Image:
The name refers to this point's location in the depression (that opens up when the jaw is relaxed) formed by the angle of the zygomatic and mandible bones.

Functions:
Dispels Wind and Cold△ and clears Heat.
> Indications: facial paralysis, trigeminal neuralgia, toothache, extremely red cheeks, deviated mouth or eye, and swelling of the jaw.

Use moxibustion with caution.

SI-19 *(tīng gōng)*
PALACE OF HEARING

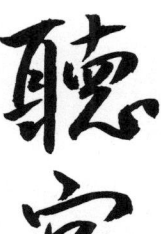

Intersecting point of the Gallbladder and Triple Burner channels on the Small Intestine channel.

With the mouth opened slightly, located in the depression between the tragus and mandibular joint.

Image:
The name refers to this point's energetic effect upon the hearing apparatus and function.

Functions:
Opens and benefits the ears and clears Heat.
> Indications: all ear disorders including deafness, tinnitus, otitis media, inflammation of the external ear canal, pus in the ear, deaf-mutism, headache due to ear pain, and aural vertigo.

Calms the Spirit.
> Indications: seizures, mania with auditory hallucinations, and melancholia.

B-1 (jīng míng)
EYE'S CLARITY

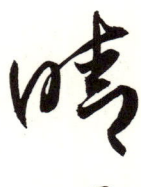
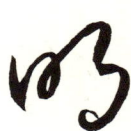

Intersecting point of the Governing, Yang-heel and Yin-heel vessels and the Small Intestine, Triple Burner and Stomach channels on the Bladder channel.

Located in the slight depression 0.1 unit superior to the inner canthus.

Image:
The name reflects the energetic function of this point on the eyes and vision. According to the classics, this point is the Intersecting point for the Yang-heel and Yin-heel vessels which greatly influence eye function.

Functions:
Opens and brightens the eyes, enriches Yin, dispels Wind, and clears Fire and Heat.

> Indications: all eye disorders including glaucomatous disorders, early-stage cataract, myopia, optic nerve atrophy, opacity of the cornea, color, night or sudden blindness, redness, tearing, itching, swelling and pain of the eye, conjunctivitis, occipital and frontal headaches, dizziness, pituitary, hypothalamus and pineal gland problems, and hysteria with vision loss.

Local effect: inner canthus pain and itching.

Moxibustion is contraindicated.

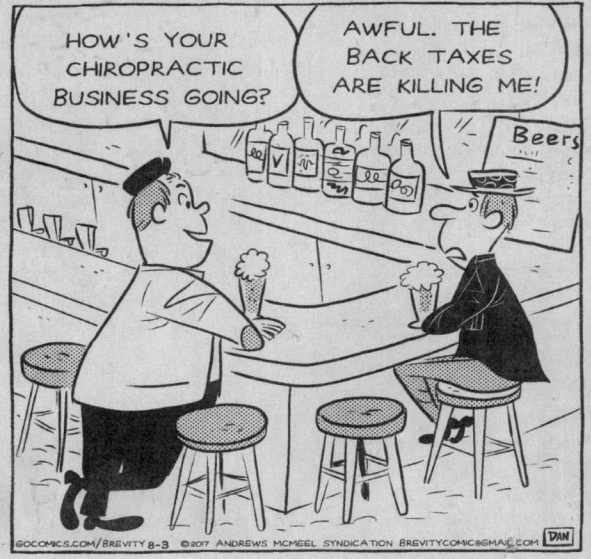

Weinfest 15th-16th

August Music Dates:
Crazy George - 12th
Bill - 11th
Mike - 26th
Eric - 19th

11am-
8am-

Always offering 12 German beers on tap. Open every day. Proudly serving the St. Croix Valley since 1999. Visit - Midi Restaurant @ Cella Vinaria Wine Bar in Duluth
Check out our new website!
www.winzerstuberestaurant.com
715-381-5092 $$

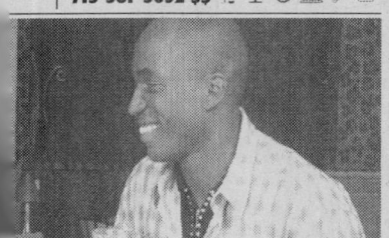
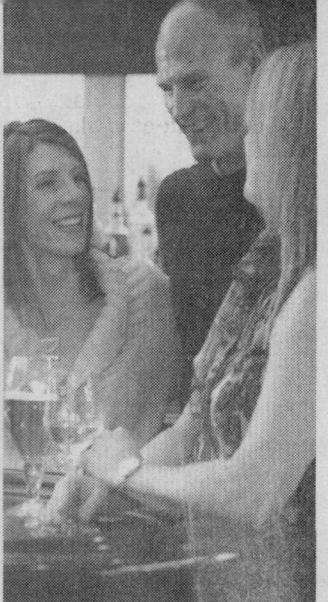

B-2 (zăn zhú)
COLLECTION OF BAMBOO

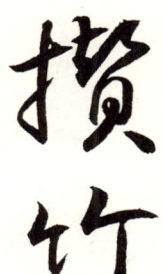

Located superior to B-1 on the medial end of the eyebrow.

Image:
The name refers to this point's location near the eyebrows, which resemble a collection of bamboo leaves.

Functions:
Opens and brightens the eyes, dispels Wind and Cold,△ and clears Heat.
> Indications: hysteria with vision loss, all eye disorders including myopia, optic nerve atrophy, hyperthyroidism with protruding eyes, color or night blindness, redness, tearing, itching, swelling and pain of the eye, conjunctivitis, blurred vision, eyelid spasms, frontal headache, dizziness, facial paralysis, and trigeminal neuralgia.

Clears the nose.
> Indications: various nasal disorders including rhinitis, sinusitis, and hay fever.

Strengthens the back.
> Indications: acute lower back injuries with muscular spasm, inflammation, motor impairment or paralysis.

Local effect: pain in the supraorbital region.

Use moxibustion with caution.

B-7 (tōng tiān)
PENETRATING HEAVEN

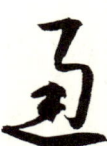

Located 1 unit anterior and 1.5 units lateral to GV-20.

Image:
The name refers to the channel Qi which penetrates and communicates with the highest reaches of "heaven" (the crown of the head), particularly GV-20. Also, *tong tian* was the name of a hat that was fastened to the head over this point.

Functions:
Clears the nose, dispels Wind, Wind-Cold,△ and Wind-Heat.

> Indications: hysteria, facial paralysis, hemiplegia, headache, pain and heaviness of the vertex of the head, dizziness, nasal discharge, epistaxis, sinusitis, and rhinorrhea.

B-10 (tiān zhù)
HEAVEN'S PILLAR

Located about 1.3 units lateral to GV-15, on the lateral border of the trapezius muscle.

Image:
The name refers to this point's location near the upper cervical region and the surrounding muscle which supports the head or "heaven" like a pillar.

Functions:
Opens the sensory orifices, dispels Wind, Wind-Cold,$^\triangle$ Wind-Heat, Wind-Phlegm and Cold,$^\triangle$ reduces fever, and clears Heat.

> Indications: asthma, neurasthenia, sensation of heaviness of the head, fever, dizziness, eye pain and inflammation, dim vision, nasal congestion, inability to smell, and throat pain and swelling.

Strengthens or relaxes the sinews and strengthens the back.

> Indications: Cold-predominant painful obstruction, childhood convulsions, seizures, ataxia, occipital headache, whiplash and traumatic neck injuries, neck stiffness, difficult breathing and chest pain, back pain, and lower extremity weakness.

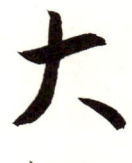

B-11 (dà zhù)
GREAT SHUTTLE

Sea of Blood point, Influential point of the bones, Intersecting point of the Small Intestine channel on the Bladder channel.

Located 1.5 units lateral to the lower border of the spinous process of the first thoracic vertebra (GV-13).

Image:
The name suggests a weaving action, referring to this point's effect on the bones and joints. It may also refer to the prominent first thoracic vertebra's spinous process.

Functions:
Regulates the Lungs, diffuses Lung Qi, expands and relaxes the chest, dispels Wind, Wind-Cold,△ Wind-Heat and Cold,△ clears Heat, and facilitates Blood flow.

> Indications: malarial disorders, pneumonia, bronchitis, pleurisy, common cold, tidal fever, high fever and chills with no sweating, dizziness, chest and flank distention, shortness of breath, cough, sore throat, and dysphonia.

Relaxes the sinews, benefits the joints, and strengthens the bones.

> Indications: atrophy syndrome, arthritis, childhood convulsions, various joint problems including painful obstruction with joint deformity, neck and spinal pain and stiffness.

Local effect: soreness and pain of the interscapular region.

B-12 (fēng mén)
WIND'S GATE

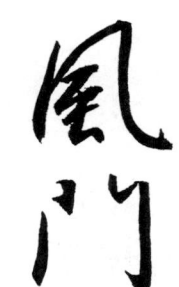

Intersecting point of the Governing vessel on the Bladder channel.

Located 1.5 units lateral to the lower border of the spinous process of the second thoracic vertebra.

Image:
The name describes the importance of this point in regulating and dispersing external pathogenic Wind that has entered or gathered here.

Functions:
Regulates the Lungs (especially Qi), diffuses Lung Qi, expands and relaxes the chest, dispels Wind, Wind-Cold,[△] Wind-Heat and Cold,[△] transforms Phlegm-Cold,[△] alleviates exterior conditions, and stimulates sweating.

   Indications: pulmonary tuberculosis, pneumonia, common cold, bronchitis, pleurisy, asthma, urticaria, fever and chills, headache, neck stiffness, cough, whooping cough, vomiting, chest and back pain, and dyspnea.

Clears the nose.

   Indications: all nasal disorders including sneezing, nasal congestion with discharge, and epistaxis.

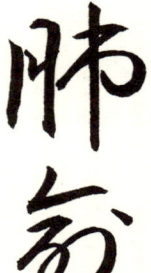

B-13 *(fèi shū)*
LUNG'S HOLLOW

Associated point of the Lung.

Located 1.5 units lateral to the lower border of the spinous process of the third thoracic vertebra (GV-12).

Image:
The name refers to this point's regulation of the Lungs. *Hollow* suggests a container or conveyor through which the circulating Qi of the Organ passes. Hollow points can both reflect and treat Organ disharmony. Not all hollow points are associated with the Organs, but may also be associated with channels (B-14 *[jue yin shu]*) or tissues (B-17 *[ge shu]*).

Functions:
Regulates and tonifies the Lung (especially Qi), regulates the upper Burner, tonifies ancestral Qi, diffuses Lung Qi, expands and relaxes the chest, dispels Wind, Wind-Cold,△ Wind-Dryness, Wind-Heat and Cold,△ transforms Phlegm, Phlegm-Cold,△ Damp-Phlegm and Phlegm-Heat, clears Heat, releases exterior conditions, and stimulates sweating.

> Indications: upper Burner-wasting and thirsting syndrome, steaming bone syndrome, atrophy syndrome due to Lung Heat, insanity, convulsions, Lung Abscess, pulmonary tuberculosis, pleurisy, asthma, bronchitis, urticaria, tidal fever, spontaneous sweating, night sweats, insomnia, cough, hemoptysis, neck and back stiffness, and lower back pain.

Redirects rebellious Qi downward.

> Indications: painful obstruction of the throat, chest fullness with difficult breathing, and vomiting.

B-14 *(jué yīn shū)*
ABSOLUTE YIN HOLLOW

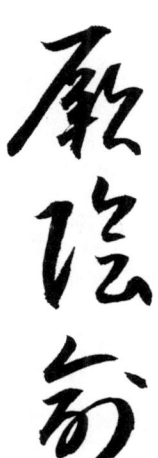

Associated point of the Pericardium.

Located 1.5 units lateral to the lower border of the spinous process of the fourth thoracic vertebra.

Image:
The name refers to this point's relationship to the Absolute Yin channels of the Pericardium and Liver. *Hollow* suggests a container or conveyor through which the circulating Qi passes (see B-13 *[fei shu]*).

Functions:
Regulates and tonifies the Heart (especially Qi and Yang) and expands and relaxes the chest.

Indications: rheumatic heart disease, neurasthenia, intercostal neuralgia, chest pain, anxiety and palpitations, stifling sensation in the chest, cough, and dyspnea.

Spreads Liver Qi and redirects rebellious Qi downward.

Indications: chest, hypochondriac and epigastric pain due to stagnant Liver Qi, melancholia, vomiting, and hiccups.

B-15 (xīn shū)
HEART'S HOLLOW

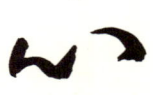
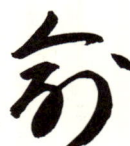

Associated point of the Heart channel.

Located 1.5 units lateral to the lower border of the spinous process of the fifth thoracic vertebra (GV-11).

Image:
The name refers to this point's relationship to the Heart. *Hollow* suggests a container or conveyor through which the circulating Qi passes (see B-13 *[fei shu]*).

Functions:
Regulates and tonifies the Heart (especially Qi, Yang and Blood), regulates the upper Burner, tonifies ancestral Qi, clears Heart Fire and Heat, cools Heat in the Blood, transforms Heart Phlegm, and expands and relaxes the chest.

> Indications: menopausal syndrome, pulmonary tuberculosis, rheumatic heart disease, neurasthenia, mutism, night sweats, fever and chills, cough with or without blood, epistaxis, chest pain with irritability and depression, chest pain penetrating to the upper back, and sensation of heat in the palms and soles.

Calms the Spirit, strengthens and clears the Brain, and transforms Wind-Phlegm.

> Indications: seizures, mania, hysteria, hallucinations, depression, forgetfulness, disorientation, dream-disturbed sleep, insomnia, anxiety and palpitations, and nocturnal emission.

B-16 (dū shū)
GOVERNING HOLLOW

Located 1.5 units lateral to the lower border of the spinous process of the sixth thoracic vertebra (GV-10).

Image:
The name refers to this point's relationship to the Governing vessel, particularly its ability to drain excess or stagnation from the channel. *Hollow* suggests a container or conveyor through which the circulating Qi passes (see B-13 *[fei shu]*).

Functions:
Expands and relaxes the chest, benefits the diaphragm, clears Heat, and cools Heat in the Blood.
> Indications: pericarditis, endocarditis, psoriasis, chest pain, diaphragmatic spasms, abdominal distention and pain, fever and chills, boils, and abscesses.

Facilitates lactation.
> Indications: mastitis.

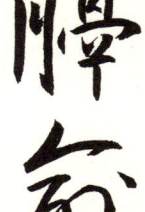

B-17 (gé shū)
DIAPHRAGM'S HOLLOW

Influential point of the Blood.

Located 1.5 units lateral to the lower border of the spinous process of the seventh thoracic vertebra (GV-9).

Image:
The name refers to this point's relationship to the diaphragm. *Hollow* suggests a container or conveyor through which the circulating Qi passes (see B-13 *[fei shu]*).

Functions:
Regulates and tonifies the Spleen (especially Qi), regulates and tonifies the Blood, nourishes Dry Blood, clears Heat, cools Heat in the Blood, invigorates the Blood, generates Fluids, facilitates Blood flow, and enriches Yin.

> Indications: upper Burner-wasting and thirsting syndrome with intense thirst, steaming bone syndrome, various skin disorders including scrofula, urticaria, psoriasis, abscesses and carbuncles, anemia, amenorrhea due to Blood Dryness, tidal fever, fever and chills, night sweats, excessive sweating, stomachache due to Blood stasis, abdominal distention and lumps, lassitude, and chronic somnolence.

Benefits the diaphragm.

> Indications: various diaphragmatic disorders including hiatus hernia, diaphragmatic spasms, and esophageal constriction.

Contains the Blood.△

> Indications: all chronic bleeding including epistaxis and hemoptysis.

B-18 (gān shū)
LIVER'S HOLLOW

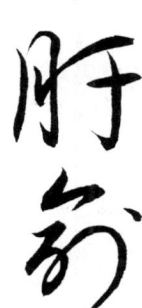

Associated point of the Liver.

Located 1.5 units lateral to the lower border of the spinous process of the ninth thoracic vertebra (GV-8).

Image:
The name refers to this point's relationship to the Liver. *Hollow* suggests a container or conveyor through which the circulating Qi passes (see B-13 *[fei shu]*).

Functions:
Regulates and tonifies the Liver (especially Qi, Yang and Blood), subdues Liver Yang, regulates the Gallbladder, transforms Damp-Heat (especially Liver and Gallbladder), regulates Qi, and facilitates Qi flow.

> Indications: insanity, seizures, muscular tetany, atrophy syndrome, jaundice, hepatitis and cholecystitis due to Damp-Heat, pancreatitis, dizziness and vertigo due to Liver Yang excess, chronic fatigue, reduced appetite, chest and abdominal fullness and distention, and sciatica.

Brightens the eyes.

> Indications: all eye disorders including myopia, conjunctivitis, blurred vision, night blindness, optic nerve atrophy, and redness of the inner canthus.

Clears Liver Fire, Heat and cools Heat in the Blood.

> Indications: hemoptysis or epistaxis due to Liver Fire, tidal fever, headache, abnormal uterine bleeding, insomnia, and dream-disturbed sleep.

Spreads Liver Qi.
> Indications: intercostal neuralgia or hypochondriac pain due to stagnant Liver Qi, neurasthenia, amenorrhea, irregular menstruation, disorientation, and irritability.

Regulates the Stomach.
> Indications: gastritis, epigastric and abdominal pain.

Softens hard masses.
> Indications: scrofula, cirrhosis of the liver or enlarged liver.

B-19 (dǎn shū)
GALLBLADDER'S HOLLOW

Associated point of the Gallbladder.
Located 1.5 units lateral to the lower border of the spinous process of the tenth thoracic vertebra (GV-7).

Image:
The name refers to this point's relationship to the Gallbladder. *Hollow* suggests a container or conveyor through which the circulating Qi passes (see B-13 *[fei shu]*).

Functions:
Regulates the Liver (especially Qi and Yang) and Gallbladder, clears Liver Fire and Heat, transforms Damp-Heat (especially Liver and Gallbladder), and regulates Qi.

    Indications: pulmonary tuberculosis, jaundice, hepatitis, pleurisy, pancreatitis, cholecystitis, insomnia, dream-disturbed sleep, intermittent fever and headache, sore throat, bitter taste in the mouth, pain in the chest, back, costal and hypochondriac regions.

Brightens the eyes.

    Indications: various eye disorders including myopia, conjunctivitis, and optic nerve atrophy.

Expels parasites.

    Indications: roundworms in the bile ducts and intestines.

Regulates the Stomach (especially the Qi).

    Indications: gastritis, and epigastric and abdominal distention.

Softens hard masses.

    Indications: scrofula and axillary lymphadenitis.

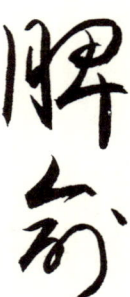

B-20 (pí shū)
SPLEEN'S HOLLOW

Associated point of the Spleen.
Located 1.5 units lateral to the lower border of the spinous process of the eleventh thoracic vertebra (GV-6).

Image:
The name refers to this point's relationship to the Spleen. *Hollow* suggests a container or conveyor through which the circulating Qi passes (see B-13 *[fei shu]*).

Functions:
Regulates, strengthens and tonifies the Spleen (especially Qi and Yang), regulates the Stomach (especially Qi and Yin) and middle Burner, nourishes Blood Dryness, tonifies nutritive Qi and Blood, reduces digestive stagnation, warms Cold,^△ transforms Dampness, Damp-Heat (especially Spleen and Stomach), Damp-Phlegm and Phlegm-Cold,^△ and dries Dampness^△ and Damp-Cold.^△

> Indications: middle Burner-wasting and thirsting syndrome, atrophy syndrome due to Damp-Heat, Qi-type painful urinary dysfunction, dysenteric disorders, Yin-type jaundice, hepatitis, neurasthenia, ascites, gastritis, enteritis, pancreatitis, ulcers, stomachache or epigastric pain due to Stomach Qi deficiency and Cold, lack of appetite, indigestion, borborygmus, abdominal distention and pain, edema, stomach dysfunction with insomnia, urticaria, anxiety and palpitations due to Qi and Blood deficiency, anemia, dizziness and vertigo due to Phlegm, esophageal constriction, vomiting, cough with profuse sputum, acute or chronic diarrhea with abdominal distention,

constipation, stool with undigested food, and extremity weakness.

Contains the Blood.△

Indications: all types of bleeding including abnormal uterine bleeding and blood in the stool.

Softens hard masses.

Indications: enlarged liver and spleen, hard abdominal masses, and lymphadenitis.

Raises middle Qi.

Indications: organ prolapse (stomach, uterovaginal, etc.).

Expedites lactation.

Indications: insufficient lactation due to deficiency.

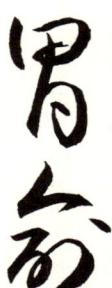

B-21 *(wèi shū)*
STOMACH'S HOLLOW

Associated point of the Stomach.

Located 1.5 units lateral to the lower border of the spinous process of the twelfth thoracic vertebra.

Image:
The name refers to this point's relationship to the Stomach. *Hollow* suggests a container or conveyor through which the circulating Qi passes (see B-13 *[fei shu]*).

Functions:
Regulates, strengthens and tonifies the Spleen (especially Qi and Yang), regulates the Stomach (especially Qi and Yin) and middle Burner, tonifies nutritive Qi, reduces digestive stagnation, clears Stomach Fire, transforms Dampness and Damp-Heat (especially Spleen and Stomach), and dries Dampness and Damp-Cold.△

> Indications: middle Burner-wasting and thirsting syndrome, dysenteric disorders, atrophy syndrome due to Damp-Heat, hepatitis, gastritis, pancreatitis, enteritis, stomachache or epigastric pain due to Stomach Qi deficiency and Cold, pain or stifling sensation in the chest and hypochondriac regions, abdominal distention and pain, loss of appetite, edema, indigestion, borborygmus, flatulence, acute or chronic diarrhea, and mid-back pain.

Redirects rebellious Qi downward.

> Indications: belching, regurgitation, vomiting, and difficulty in swallowing.

B-22 (sān jiāo shū)
TRIPLE BURNER'S HOLLOW

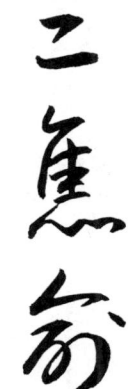

Associated point of the Triple Burner.

Located 1.5 units lateral to the lower border of the spinous process of the first lumbar vertebra (GV-5).

Image:
The name refers to this point's relationship to the Triple Burner. *Hollow* suggest a container or conveyor through which the circulating Qi passes (see B-13 *[fei shu]*).

Functions:
Regulates the Triple Burner and Water Pathways, tonifies the Kidneys (especially Yang), and resolves Dampness.

    Indications: dysenteric disorders, acute or chronic nephritis, painful urinary dysfunction, ascites, neurasthenia, anxiety and palpitations due to congested Fluids, edema, emaciation, dizziness and headache, vomiting, abdominal distention, indigestion, borborygmus, diarrhea, urinary retention, urinary incontinence, back and shoulder muscle spasms and stiffness.

Expels stones (especially urinary tract).

    Indications: kidney stones.

B-23 (shèn shū)
KIDNEY'S HOLLOW

Associated point of the Kidney.
Located 1.5 units lateral to the lower border of the spinous process of the second lumbar vertebra (GV-4).

Image:
The name refers to this point's relationship to the Kidney. *Hollow* suggests a container or conveyor through which the circulating Qi passes (see B-13 *[fei shu]*).

Functions:
Tonifies the Kidneys (especially Qi and Yang) and Essence,$^\triangle$ regulates the lower Burner, warms the Yang$^\triangle$ and Cold,$^\triangle$ and tonifies source Qi.

> Indications: lower Burner-wasting and thirsting syndrome, atrophy syndrome due to deficiency, infantile paralysis, pulmonary tuberculosis with chills and shortness of breath, asthma, bronchial asthma, neurasthenia, anemia, generalized weakness, hair loss, seizures, menopausal syndrome, irregular menstruation, amenorrhea, dysmenorrhea, leukorrhea, impotence, genital pain, abdominal cramps, and diarrhea with undigested food.

Regulates Water Pathways, promotes urination, and resolves Dampness.

> Indications: diabetes, chronic nephritis, prostatitis, painful urinary dysfunction, urinary tract infection, urinary incontinence, blood in the urine, and urinary retention and edema.

Benefits the ears and brightens the eyes.

Indications: deafness, diminished hearing, tinnitus, blurred and dim vision, eye fatigue, and optic nerve atrophy.

Stabilizes Kidney Qi$^\triangle$ and strengthens the lower back and knees.

Indications: premature ejaculation, spermatorrhea, urinary incontinence, emaciation and weakness, cold and weakness, and chronic knee, sacral or lower back pain.

Expels stones (especially urinary tract).

Indications: kidney stones.

Strengthens the Brain.$^\triangle$

Indications: forgetfulness, disorientation, poor concentration, lethargy, and sensation of heaviness of the head.

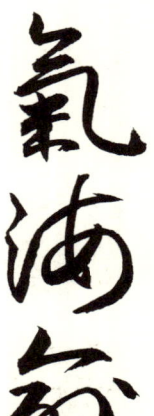

B-24 *(qì hǎi shū)*
SEA OF QI'S HOLLOW

Located 1.5 units lateral to the lower border of the spinous process of the third lumbar vertebra.

Image:
The name refers to this point's relationship to CV-6 *(qi hai)* and to its usefulness in regulating the Qi and Blood within the "cinnabar field" (see CV-5). *Hollow* suggests a container or conveyor through which the circulating Qi passes (see B-13 *[fei shu]*).

Functions:
Strengthens the lower back and regulates Qi and Blood.
> Indications: irregular menstruation, dysmenorrhea, functional uterine bleeding, lower back pain and stiffness, and lower extremity paralysis.

B-25 (dà cháng shū)
LARGE INTESTINE'S HOLLOW

Associated point of the Large Intestine.

Located 1.5 units lateral to the lower border of the spinous process of the fourth lumbar vertebra (GV-3).

Image:
The name refers to this point's relationship to the Large Intestine. *Hollow* suggests a container or conveyor through which the circulating Qi passes (see B-13 *[fei shu]*).

Functions:
Regulates and moistens the Intestines, resolves Damp-Heat (especially Large Intestine), warms Cold,$^\triangle$ and dries Damp-Cold$^\triangle$ (especially Large Intestine).

    Indications: dysenteric disorders, childhood nutritional impairment, all intestinal disorders including acute intestinal obstruction and enteritis, appendicitis, borborygmus, flatulence, abdominal pain and distention, abdominal masses, and stabbing pain around the umbilicus, difficult or painful defecation or urination, constipation, diarrhea, rectal prolapse, and hemorrhoids.

Strengthens the lower back.

    Indications: lower back pain and stiffness, and sciatica.

B-26 (guān yuán shū)
HINGE AT THE SOURCE HOLLOW

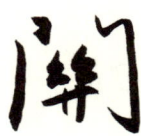
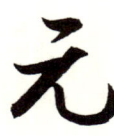

Located 1.5 units lateral to the lower border of the spinous process of the fifth lumbar vertebra.

Image:
The name refers to this point's relationship to Hinge at the Source (CV-4 [guan yuan]) and the surrounding area. *Hollow* suggests a container or conveyor through which the circulating Qi passes (see B-13 [fei shu]).

Functions:
Regulates and moistens the Intestines, regulates the lower Burner, resolves Dampness and Damp-Heat, warms Cold,^△ and dries Damp-Cold.^△

>Indications: lower Burner-wasting and thirsting syndrome, dysenteric disorders, painful urinary dysfunction, chronic peritonitis or enteritis, abdominal distention and pain, cystitis, urinary incontinence, constipation, diarrhea, and hemorrhoids.

Strengthens the lower back and knees.

>Indications: lower back pain and stiffness, sciatica, and lower limb paralysis.

B-27 (xiǎo cháng shū)
SMALL INTESTINE'S HOLLOW

Associated point of the Small Intestine.

Located 1.5 units lateral to the posterior midline of the back, level with the first posterior sacral foramen (B-31).

Image:
The name refers to this point's relationship to the Small Intestine. *Hollow* suggests a container or conveyor through which the circulating Qi passes (see B-13 *[fei shu]*).

Functions:
Regulates and moistens the Intestines, resolves Dampness and Damp-Heat (especially lower Burner).

    Indications: dysenteric disorders with pus and blood, enteritis, peritonitis, urethritis, colic, lower abdominal pain and distention, leukorrhea, constipation, hemorrhoids, and foot swelling.

Strengthens the lower back.

    Indications: lower back, sacral or sacroiliac pain and stiffness, and sciatica.

Regulates the Water Pathways and stabilizes the Essence.

    Indications: dysuria, urinary incontinence, blood in the urine, and urination with seminal discharge.

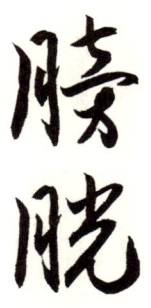

B-28 (páng guāng shū)
BLADDER'S HOLLOW

Associated point of the Bladder.

Located 1.5 units lateral to the posterior midline of the back, level with the second posterior sacral foramen (B-32).

Image:
The name refers to this point's relationship to the Bladder. *Hollow* suggests a container or conveyor through which the circulating Qi passes (see B-13 *[fei shu]*).

Functions:
Regulates the Bladder and Water Pathways, clears Heat, and resolves Damp-Heat (especially Bladder).
> Indications: painful urinary dysfunction, prostatitis, urinary incontinence, urination with seminal discharge, urinary tract infection, blood in the urine, spermatorrhea, genital swelling and pain, borborygmus, lower abdominal pain and distention, constipation, and diarrhea.

Strengthens the lower back.
> Indications: lower back, sacral or sacroiliac pain and stiffness, sciatica, and cold back and lower extremities.

Expels stones (especially urinary tract).
> Indications: lower urinary tract stones.

B-29 *(zhōng lǚ shū)*
CENTRAL SPINE HOLLOW

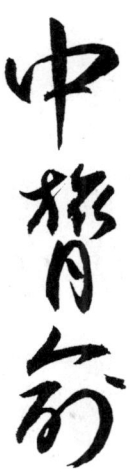

Located 1.5 units lateral to the posterior midline of the back, level with the third posterior sacral foramen (B-33).

Image:
The name refers to this point's relationship to the entire vertebral column. *Hollow* suggests a container or conveyor through which the circulating Qi passes (see B-13 *[fei shu]*).

Functions:
Strengthens the back, dispels Wind and Cold.△

Indications: pain on both sides of the spine from the neck to the sacrum, spinal pain and stiffness, sciatica, lower back pain, and groin pain due to hernia.

B-30 *(bái huán shū)*
WHITE RING HOLLOW

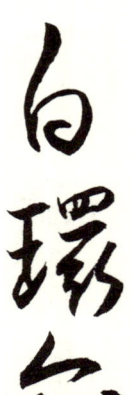

Located 1.5 units lateral to the posterior midline of the back, level with the fourth posterior sacral foramen (B-34).

Image:
The name refers to this point's relationship to the sphincter muscles (particularly the anus, and to a lesser extent the bladder). *White ring* suggests the shape of the muscle. *Hollow* suggests a container or conveyor through which the circulating Qi passes (see B-13 *[fei shu]*).

Functions:
Stabilizes Essence△ and lower orifices,△ transforms Damp-Heat (especially lower Burner).

> Indications: various anal disorders including anal cramps, leukorrhea, spermatorrhea, uterovaginal inflammation, urinary incontinence due to paralysis, excessive uterine bleeding, painful defecation or urination and constipation with painful defecation, sciatica, lower back, sacral or coccygeal pain, and lower extremity weakness.

B-31~34 (bā liáo)
EIGHT FORAMINA

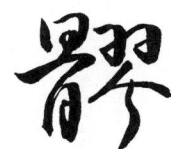

Located within the four sacral foramina.

Image:
The name refers to a group of points located bilaterally in the sacral foramina: B-31 (upper foramen), B-32 (second foramen), B-33 (middle foramen), and B-34 (lower foramen). Their similar functions explain their classification as a group.

Functions:
Regulates the lower Burner and menstruation, transforms Damp-Heat (especially lower Burner), stabilizes Essence,△ invigorates the Blood, and promotes urination.

    Indications: infertility, impotence, irregular menstruation, dysmenorrhea, ovarian pain or inflammation, leukorrhea, spermatorrhea, orchitis, urinary retention, difficult urination due to infection, skin irritation in the genital region, uterovaginal inflammation, peritonitis, diarrhea, and constipation.

Strengthens the lower back.

    Indications: lower back and foot numbness, lower extremity paralysis, pain and stiffness of the lower back and sacrum, and sciatica.

Redirects Qi upward.

    Indications: anal fissures, hemorrhoids, and uterovaginal prolapse.

Expedites labor.

    Indications: difficult or delayed labor.

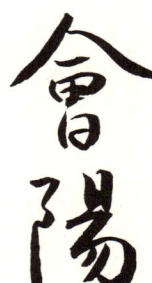

B-35 *(huì yáng)*
MEETING OF YANG

Beside the inferior tip of the coccyx, located 0.5 unit lateral to the posterior midline of the back.

Image:
The name refers to this point's location next to GV-1, where the Yang Qi tends to gather at the base of the spine. CV-1 *(hui yin)*, or "Meeting of Yin," complements this point.

Functions:
Clears Heat and transforms Damp-Heat (especially lower Burner).
> Indications: dysenteric disorders, lower back pain due to menstruation, leukorrhea, impotence, genital sweating, hemorrhoids, coccygeal pain, and diarrhea.

B-36 *(chéng fú)*
BEARING SUPPORT

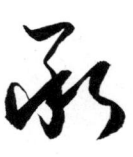

Located at the midpoint of the transverse gluteal fold.

Image:
The name suggests this point's anatomical and functional support of the trunk and upper body.

Functions:
Strengthens the lower back and facilitates Qi flow.
  Indications: anal, coccygeal, genital, lower back or gluteal pain and inflammation, sciatica, lower extremity paralysis, hemorrhoids, and constipation.

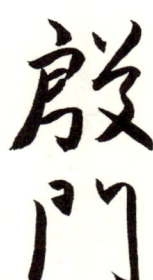

B-37 (yīn mén)
ABUNDANCE GATE

Located 6 units inferior to B-36 on a line connecting B-36 and B-40.

Image:
The name suggests a "gateway" which influences the abundant musculature (nourished by Qi and Blood) around this point.

Functions:
Strengthens the lower back and relaxes the sinews.
> Indications: infantile paralysis, inability to bend the back or lie prone, pain and stiffness of the hip, lower back and thigh, sciatica, paralysis of the hip extensor and knee flexor muscles, and herniated lumbar disc.

B-39 *(wěi yáng)*
ENTRUSTING YANG

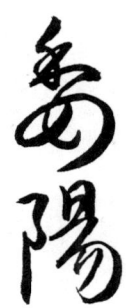

Lower Sea point of the Triple Burner channel.

Located level and lateral to B-40 on the medial side of the tendon of the biceps femoris muscle.

Image:
Entrusting refers to this point's duty of regulating the Yang Qi which gathers here. *Yang* further suggests this point's position lateral (the Yang side) to B-40.

Functions:
Regulates the Triple Burner, Bladder and Water Pathways, promotes urination, and resolves Damp-Heat.

> Indications: painful urinary dysfunction, nephritis, stifling sensation in the chest and hypochondrium, abdominal distention, lower back pain extending to the abdomen, dysuria, chyluria, urinary tract infection, urinary retention or incontinence, constipation, and hemorrhoids.

Local effect: knee pain and stiffness, numbness or muscle spasm of the lower extremities.

B-40 (wěi zhōng)
ENTRUSTING MIDDLE

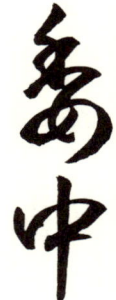

Sea and Earth point of the Bladder channel.

Midpoint of the transverse crease of the popliteal fossa, located between the tendons of the biceps femoris and semitendinosis muscles.

Image:
Entrusting suggests this point's duty of regulating the middle Qi which gathers here. *Middle* corresponds to its classification as an Earth point and refers to its location on the popliteal fossa.

Functions:
Dispels Wind, clears Heat and Summerheat,° cools Heat in the Blood,° transforms Damp-Heat (especially Bladder and Intestines) and Damp-Summerheat, alleviates pain, and calms the Fetus.

> Indications: erysipelas or ulceration due to Damp-Heat, restless fetus disorder due to Heat in the Blood, malarial disorders, herpes zoster, tidal fever, fever without sweating, spontaneous sweating, carbuncles, boils, vomiting, epistaxis, twisting pain in the chest and abdomen, acute abdominal pain, urinary incontinence, dysuria, and diarrhea.

Strengthens the lower back, benefits the hips, strengthens the knees, and relaxes the sinews.

> Indications: muscular tetany, convulsions, hemiplegia, all knee joint diseases, gastrocnemius muscle spasms, hip joint pain and restricted movement, lower extremity paralysis or atrophy, lower back pain, and sciatica.

Revives consciousness.

Indications: Heatstroke and coma due to stroke.

Use moxibustion with caution.

B-42 (pò hù)
ANIMAL SOUL DOOR

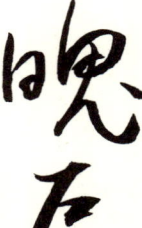

Located 3 units lateral to the lower border of the spinous process of the third thoracic vertebra (GV-12).

Image:
The name refers to this point's governance over the *po* or animal soul which resides in the Lungs. *Po* is associated with passion, instinct and attachment or Yin movement directed toward earth, which restricts or holds back the *hun* or spiritual soul (see B-47 [*hun men*]). *Door* suggests an entrance.

Functions:
Regulates the Lungs, diffuses Lung Qi, and redirects rebellious Qi downward.

> Indications: pulmonary tuberculosis, bronchitis, pleurisy, asthma, stifling sensation in the chest, shoulder and back pain, neck stiffness, cough with profuse sputum, and vomiting.

B-43 (gāo huāng shū)
FATTY VITAL HOLLOW

Located 3 units lateral to the lower border of the spinous process of the fourth thoracic vertebra.

Image:
The name refers to this point's relationship to the innermost part of the body, thought to be the fatty tissue between the Heart and diaphragm. According to the ancients, diseases which settle in this area are almost beyond cure (*bing ru gao huang*). Classical texts state that it effectively treats chronic conditions which do not respond to conventional treatment. In addition, Taoists claimed that proper use of this point produced immortality, which overstates the preventive attributes of this point. *Hollow* suggests a container or conveyor through which circulating Qi passes (see B-13 *[fei shu]*). Some modern texts simply call this point *gao huang*.

Functions:
Regulates the Lungs (especially Qi), expands and relaxes the chest, regulates and tonifies Qi and Blood,$^\triangle$ moistens Dryness, transforms Phlegm and Phlegm-Cold,$^\triangle$ and redirects rebellious Qi downward.

　Indications: pulmonary tuberculosis, bronchitis, asthma, Lung Abscess, dry skin, dizziness, vomiting, cough, and hiccups.

Tonifies the Kidneys (especially Yang and Yin)$^\triangle$ and warms the Yang$^\triangle$.

　Indications: chronic consumptive disorders due to deficiency, generalized weakness due to prolonged illness, neurasthenia, nocturnal emission, and night sweats.

Calms the Spirit, restores collapsed Yang,^△ regulates and tonifies the Heart (especially Qi).

Indications: mania, depression, insomnia, anxiety and palpitations, forgetfulness, and chest pain.

Local effect: frozen shoulder, muscular pain of the shoulder and back.

B-44 *(shén táng)*
SPIRIT'S HALL

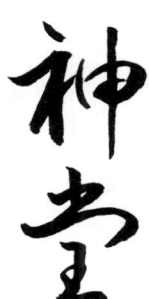

Located 3 units lateral to the lower border of the spinous process of the fifth thoracic vertebra (GV-11).

Image:

The name refers to this point's governance over the *shen* or Spirit, which resides in the Heart. *Shen* is primarily associated with the integrative functions of consciousness. Considered the unifying force or essential spirit, *shen* harmonizes the other Organ spirits: *po, hun, yi* and *zhi* (see B-42 *[po hu]*, B-47 *[hun men]*, B-49 *[yi she]*, and B-52 *[zhi shi]* respectively). *Tang* is a hall or court of law, suggesting a place of residence or governance.

Functions:

Regulates the Heart (especially Qi), expands and relaxes the chest, and clears Heat.

    Indications: various heart disorders, asthma, bronchitis, stifling sensation in the chest, palpitations, chest pain, fever and chills, and cough.

Calms the Spirit and clears the Brain.

    Indications: mania, hysteria, depression, disorientation, anxiety and palpitations, and restlessness.

Local effect: spasms and contracture of the upper back muscles, shoulder and back pain.

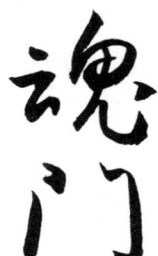

B-47 *(hún mén)*
SPIRITUAL SOUL GATE

Located 3 units lateral to the lower border of the spinous process of the ninth thoracic vertebra (GV-8).

Image:
The name refers to this point's governance over the *hun* or spiritual soul, which resides in the Liver. *Hun* is associated with intuition, imagination and higher consciousness or Yang movement directed upward toward heaven. When cultivated, it transcends the influence of *po* (see B-42 *[po hu]*). *Gate* suggests an entrance.

Functions:
Regulates the Liver (especially Qi and Yang), spreads Liver Qi, and clears Heat.

    Indications: hypertension, pleurisy, jaundice, neurasthenia, headache, distending pain in the chest and hypochondrium, and mid-back pain and stiffness.

Redirects rebellious Qi downward and regulates the Stomach (especially Qi).

    Indications: vomiting, dizziness, difficulty in swallowing food, borborygmus, and stomachache.

B-49 (yì shè)
INTELLIGENCE LODGE

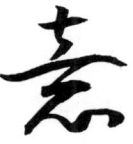

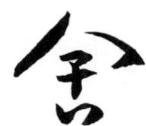

Located 3 units lateral to the lower border of the spinous process of the eleventh thoracic vertebra (GV-11).

Image:
The name refers to this point's governance over the *yi* or intelligence, which resides in the Spleen. *Yi* is associated with the cognitive, reflective, and organizational processes of the mind. *Lodge* denotes a place of residence.

Functions:
Regulates and strengthens the Spleen (especially Qi and Yang), regulates the Stomach (especially Qi), transforms Dampness and Damp-Heat, and redirects rebellious Qi downward.

> Indications: middle Burner-wasting and thirsting syndrome, jaundice, nausea, vomiting, belching and regurgitation, lack of appetite, epigastric and abdominal pain and distention, borborygmus, diarrhea, and back pain.

B-52 (zhì shì)
WILL'S CHAMBER

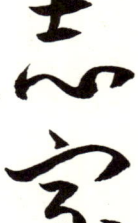

Located 3 units lateral to the lower border of the spinous process of the second lumbar vertebra (GV-4).

Image:
The name refers to this point's governance over the *zhi* or will, which resides in the Kidneys. *Zhi*, which is intimately connected with the Essence, is associated with individual intention, ambition or aspiration. *Chamber* refers to a place of residence.

Functions:
Tonifies the Kidney (especially Kidney Qi, Yang and Yin), Essence△ and source Qi,△ stabilizes Kidney Qi, regulates the Water Pathways, and resolves Dampness.

> Indications: painful urinary dysfunction, infertility, impotence, prostatitis, nephritis, anemia, edema, nausea, vomiting, spasmodic pain in the hypochondrium, epigastric fullness and pain, lower back pain and stiffness, swelling of the perineum or sexual organs, scrotal eczema, nocturnal emission, urinary tract infection, urinary incontinence, dysuria, and diarrhea.

B-54 *(zhì biān)*
ORDER'S FRONTIER

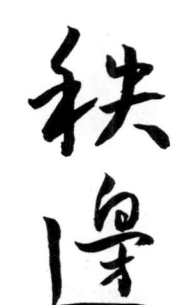

Located 3 units lateral to the posterior midline of the back level with the hiatus of the sacrum.

Image:
The name refers to this point's location at the end of the orderly column of Bladder channel points.

Functions:
Strengthens the lower back and resolves Damp-Heat (especially lower Burner).

> Indications: gluteal, lower back and sacral pain, sciatica, paralysis of the hip extensor muscles and the lower extremities, hemorrhoids, prostatitis, difficult urination or defecation, and genital pain.

B-57 (chéng shān)
SUPPORTING MOUNTAIN

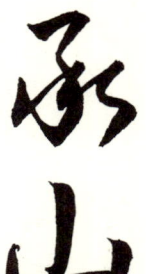

Located directly inferior to the belly of the gastrocnemius muscle on the line connecting B-40 and the tendon calcaneus, approximately 8 units below B-40.

Image:
The name refers to this point's location at the base of the muscular relief or "mountain" (the belly of the gastrocnemius muscle).

Functions:
Relaxes the sinews, strengthens the lower back, dispels Wind, and clears Heat.
> Indications: convulsions, localized muscular spasms, body tremors, lockjaw, lower back pain, lower extremity paralysis, leg Qi, and sciatica.

Regulates the Large Intestine and transforms Damp-Heat.
> Indications: hernial disorders, malarial disorders, lower body erysipelas due to Damp-Heat, urethritis, abdominal pain, anal prolapse, hemorrhoids, diarrhea, and constipation.

Local effect: gastrocnemius muscle spasm and pain.

B-58 (fēi yáng)
FLYING YANG

Connecting point of the Bladder channel.

Located 7 units directly above B-60 on the posterior border of the fibula approximately 1 unit inferior and lateral to B-57.

Image:
The name refers to this point's effectiveness against excessive, unharmonious, elevated and upward-moving (rebellious) Yang Qi.

Functions:
Dispels Wind and redirects rebellious Qi downward.

> Indications: Wind-predominant painful obstruction of the lower extremities, seizures, dizziness, headache, blurred vision, nasal obstruction, lower back pain, and sciatica.

Local effect: lower extremity and ankle joint weakness or paralysis.

B-59 (fū yáng)
TARSAL YANG

Accumulating point of the Yang-heel vessel.

Located 3 units directly above B-60 at the lateral aspect of the gastrocnemius muscle.

Image:
The name refers to this point's energetic effect upon the ankle joint articulations (tarsal bones, etc.), especially the Yang or lateral aspect of the ankle.

Functions:
Relaxes the sinews, regulates Qi, dispels Wind, and clears Heat.

> Indications: seizures, sensation of heaviness of the head, headache, hip, thigh and lower back pain with inability to stand, lower leg cramps, sciatica, leg Qi, hemmorhoids, inflammation of the ankle joint, paralysis of the plantar flexor muscles and weakness in medial deviation of the foot, and hemmorhoids.

Local effect: external malleolus pain or inflammation.

B-60 *(kūn lún)*
KUNLUN MOUNTAINS

River and Fire point of the Bladder channel.

Located in the depression between the lateral malleolus and tendocalcaneus level with the vertex of the lateral malleolus.

Image:
The name refers to this point's location next to the lateral malleolus, which resembles a mountain. The Taoists, Buddhists, and other philosophers of ancient China believed that mountains possess powerful energy and offer spiritual and physical renewal. The Kunlun mountains in China, one of the five sacred mountains to Taoists and Buddhists, are also considered the source of the Yellow River, where Chinese civilization began.

Functions:
Strengthens the back, relaxes the sinews, facilitates Qi and Blood flow, regulates the Blood, invigorates the Blood, and dispels Wind and Cold.△

> Indications: seizures, childhood convulsions, tidal fever, occipital headache, vertigo, neck, shoulder and upper back pain, spasms and stiffness, buttock, lower back and sacral pain and stiffness, lower extremity paralysis, sciatica, ankle and heel pain.

Expedites labor.

> Indications: difficult labor and lochioschesis.

Local effect: ankle and heel pain, ankle edema, and pain in the sole of the foot.

Needling is contraindicated during pregnancy.

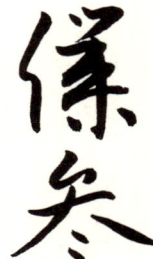

B-61 (pú cān)
SERVANT'S PARTAKING

Intersecting point of the Yang-heel vessel on the Bladder channel.

Located 1.5 units inferior to B-60 in the depression posterior and inferior to the lateral malleolus.

Image:
The name refers to this point's anatomical location, suggesting involvement or responsibility assigned to one of a lower status or position. *Can* also means "to pay respect." It is said that this part of the heel was exposed when a servant performed the ritual bow.

Functions:
Strengthens the lower back, relaxes the sinews and dispels Wind.
> Indications: seizures, muscular tetany, convulsions, muscle spasms due to severe vomiting and diarrhea, lower back pain, and knee inflammation.

Local effect: atrophy of the foot and lower leg muscles, heel pain and drop foot.

B-62 (shēn mài)
EXTENDING VESSEL

Confluent point of the Yang-heel vessel.

Located in the depression directly inferior to the external malleolus.

Image:
The name refers to this point's function as a Confluent point of the Yang-heel vessel, which extends upward to the head. *Shen* also translates as "ninth earthly branch vessel," referring to the time of day governed by the ninth earthly branch (3-5 P.M.), which corresponds to this point's channel and Organ.

Functions:
Relaxes the sinews, clears Fire and Heat, dispels Wind and Cold,△ and regulates the Yang-heel vessel.
  Indications: glaucomatous disorders, meningitis, Wind-predominant painful obstruction, daytime epileptic seizures, post-concussion syndrome, hemiplegia, voice loss due to stroke, insomnia, fatigue, dizziness, lateral and frontal headache, neck stiffness, red, painful and swollen eyes, nasal congestion and discharge, tinnitus, and uterine spasms.

Calms the Spirit.
  Indications: insanity, depression, and disorientation.

Local effect: ankle pain, weakness and cold.

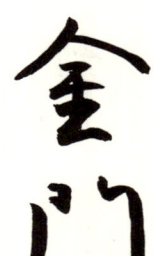

B-63 (jīn mén)
GOLDEN GATE

Accumulating point of the Bladder channel and Intersecting point of the Yang-linking vessel on the Bladder channel.

Anterior and inferior to B-62, located in the depression on the lateral aspect of the cuboid bone.

Image:
The name refers to this point's function as a source of precious Yang Qi. Gold, almost pure Yang in nature, is a Taoist symbol for incorruptibility, purity, illumination and wisdom.

Functions:
Dispels Wind and clears Heat.
> Indications: seizures, childhood convulsions, frontal headache, abdominal tension and cramps, lower back pain, and lower extremity pain and swelling.

Local effect: pain in the lateral aspect of the foot and ankle.

B-64 (jīng gǔ)
CENTRAL BONE

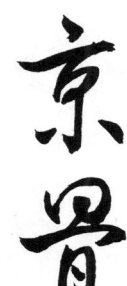

Source point of the Bladder channel.

Located posterior and inferior to the tuberosity of the fifth metatarsal bone on the junction of the red and white skin.

Image:

The name is a classical term for the tuberosity of the fifth metatarsal bone. The point is located immediately under this protuberance.

Functions:

Calms the Spirit, dispels Wind, and clears Heat.

Indications: seizures, sensation of heaviness of the head, sensation of cold in the legs, tidal fever, headache, dizziness, corneal opacity, neck stiffness, palpitations, and back pain with inability to lie supine.

B-65 (shù gǔ)
RESTRAINED BONE

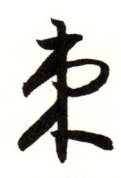
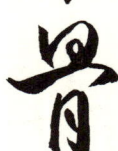

Stream and Wood point of the Bladder channel.

Located in the depression posterior and inferior to the head of the fifth metatarsal bone at the juncture of the red and white skin.

Image:
The name is a classical term for the head of the fifth metatarsal bone, this point's location. This is also the place on the foot where a shoe or sandal was fastened.

Functions:
Calms the Spirit, dispels Wind, and clears Heat.
> Indications: seizures, insanity, hysteria, convulsions, disorientation, dizziness, headache, neck stiffness, blurred vision, excessive tearing, back pain, pain in the posterior aspect of the lower extremities, and hemorrhoids.

B-66 (zú tōng gǔ)
FOOT CONNECTING VALLEY

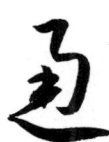
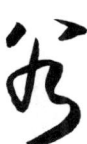

Spring and Water point of the Bladder channel.

Located in the depression anterior and inferior to the fifth metatarsophalangeal joint.

Image:
The name refers to the place where the channel Qi passes through the foot at a "valley" or depression before reaching the terminus of the channel.

Functions:
Calms the Spirit, dispels Wind, and clears Heat.
   Indications: insanity, fear, headache, vertigo, dizziness, neck stiffness, and epistaxis.

B-67 (zhì yīn)
REACHING YIN

Well and Metal point of the Bladder channel.

Located about 0.1 unit from the lateral corner of the fifth toenail.

Image:
The name refers to this point's location at the terminus of the channel on the foot where the channel Qi is approaching and about to transfer to the Kidney channel, as well as this point's influence on the deep-lying Yin energy of the Womb.

Functions:
Regulates Qi and Blood, dispels Wind, clears Heat, and transforms Damp-Heat.
> Indications: malarial disorders with no sweating, fever, melancholia, generalized body itching, parietal headache, moving pain of the chest and flanks, and sensation of heat in the soles.

Calms the Fetus and expedites labor.
> Indications: difficult labor, malposition of the fetus, and lochioschesis.

Clears the nose and brightens the eyes.
> Indications: nasal obstruction, nasal discharge, epistaxis, dim vision, and eye or medial-canthus pain.

Needling is contraindicated during pregnancy.

K-1 *(yǒng quán)*
GUSHING SPRING

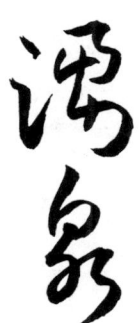

Well and Wood point of the Kidney channel.

Located in the depression produced on the sole when the foot is plantar flexed, approximately one-third the distance from the base of the second toe to the back of the heel.

Image:
The name suggests this point's fresh and active energy and refers to its location as the first point of the Kidney channel from which the channel Qi flows upward and outward like a spring or fountain.

Functions:
Tonifies the Kidneys (especially Yin) and Essence and enriches Yin.
> Indications: infertility, sensation of heat in the soles due to Kidney Yin deficiency, edema, lack of appetite, borborygmus, back pain and abdominal distention, kidney pain, constipation, diarrhea, and scrotal inflammation.

Calms the Spirit, restores collapsed Yang, revives consciousness, and transforms Heart Phlegm.
> Indications: seizures, hysteria with fainting, closed-type Wind-stroke, cardiovascular stroke, heatstroke, collapsing syndrome due to excess, convulsions, shock, asphyxia due to near drowning, high fever, and excessive sleepiness.

Clears Fire and Heat (especially the head).
> Indications: painful obstruction of the throat, hypertension, insomnia, dizziness, dry mouth and tongue, epistaxis, sore, dry or swollen throat, voice loss, and cough.

K-2 (rán gŭ)
BURNING VALLEY

Spring and Fire point of the Kidney channel.

Located in the depression on the inferior border of the tuberosity of the navicular bone.

Image:
The name describes this point's position in the depression or "valley" on the lower border of the tuberosity of the navicular bone, and its function of clearing Fire and Heat and warming Cold (this point corresponds to the fire phase). A homonym of *gu* meaning "bone" is often used with *ran gu* to refer to the classical term for the tuberosity of the navicular bone.

Functions:
Tonifies the Kidneys (especially Yang) and Essence, stabilizes Kidney Qi and Essence, clears Fire and Heat, cools Heat in the Blood, and warms Cold.△

> Indications: syrupy painful urinary dysfunction, dysenteric disorders, jaundice, cystitis, infertility, tidal fever, spontaneous sweating or night sweats, clenched jaws, irregular menstruation, uterine prolapse, impotence, spermatorrhea, itching of the genital region, and diarrhea.

Local effect: pain and swelling of the dorsal aspect of the foot.

K-3 (tài xī)
GREAT STREAM

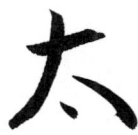
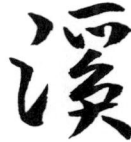

Source, Stream and Earth point of the Kidney channel.

Located in the depression between the medial malleolus and the tendocalcaneus level with the vertex of the medial malleolus.

Image:
The name refers to the channel Qi flow which, at this point, is like a majestic stream. The area between the medial malleolus and the heel tendon resembles a large stream.

Functions:
Tonifies the Kidneys (especially Qi, Yang and Yin), source Qi,△ Blood△ and Essence,△ stabilizes Kidney Qi, warms Cold,△ restores collapsed Yin, calms the Fetus, strengthens the Brain, and regulates menstruation and the Water Pathways.

> Indications: hypertension due to Kidney Yin deficiency, restless fetus disorder due to Kidney deficiency, middle and lower Burner-wasting and thirsting syndrome, chronic consumptive disorders, pulmonary tuberculosis with spermatorrhea or irregular menstruation, syrupy painful urinary dysfunction, menopausal syndrome, nephritis, renal colic, neurasthenia, headache, poor memory, tinnitus, somnolence or insomnia, lower back pain, irregular menstruation, impotence, nocturnal emission, and urinary incontinence or retention.

Enriches Yin, clears deficiency Fire and deficiency Heat, moistens Dryness, and stimulates sweating.

Indications: seizures, hypertension, painful obstruction of the throat, tonsillitis, sore throat due to deficiency Fire, trigeminal neuralgia, fever without sweating, dizziness, red eyes, toothache, asthmatic wheezing, chest mucus, chest pain, constipation, and lower extremity paralysis.

Local effect: pain in the sole of the foot.

K-4 (dà zhōng)
LARGE BELL

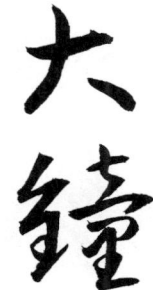

Connecting point of the Kidney channel.

Located 0.5 unit directly inferior to K-3 on the medial border of the tendocalcaneus.

Image:
The name refers to this point's location superior to the calcaneous bone on the internal heel. The internal aspect of this bone resembles a Chinese bell. A similar character (*zhong*) means "heel," suggesting an anatomical reference.

Functions:
Tonifies the Kidneys, clears deficiency Heat, and redirects rebellious Qi downward.

> Indications: asthma, chronic fatigue, vomiting, hemoptysis, dry mouth, difficulty in swallowing, chest fullness, dyspnea, abdominal distention, lower back pain and stiffness, dysuria, constipation, and painful defecation.

Calms the Spirit and clears the Brain.

> Indications: mania, hysteria with sudden laughing and crying, disorientation and depression, somnolence, and aversion to cold.

Local effect: heel pain.

K-5 (shuǐ quán)
WATER'S SPRING

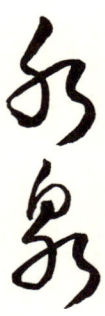

Accumulating point of the Kidney channel.

Located 1 unit directly inferior to K-3 in the depression anterior and superior to the medial side of the tuberosity of the navicular bone.

Image:
The name refers to this point's location, where the Yin or water accumulates in the channel, and suggests its classification as an Accumulating point. The name may also refer to this point's influence on urination.

Functions:
Tonifies the Kidneys and regulates the Bladder and menstruation.

> Indications: lower Burner-wasting and thirsting syndrome with frequent urination, uterine prolapse, menorrhagia, irregular menstruation, dysmenorrhea, dysuria, periumbilical pain, and blurred vision.

K-6 (zhào hăi)
LUMINOUS SEA

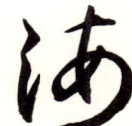

Confluent point of the Yin-heel vessel.
Located 1 unit inferior to the vertex of the medial malleolus.

Image:
The name refers to an energetic reserve or sea and this point's influence on the abdominal Sea of Qi (see CV-6 [qi hai]). In addition, *luminous* suggests the bright and clear quality of Qi found at the origin and confluence of the Yin-linking vessel.

Functions:
Tonifies the Kidneys (especially Yin), regulates the Yin-heel vessel and menstruation, clears deficiency Fire and deficiency Heat, transforms Damp-Heat, and moistens Dryness.
> Indications: hernial disorders, menopausal syndrome with Heat, neurasthenia, excessive sleepiness, edema, blurred vision or inability to keep the eyes open, medial knee injuries, uterine prolapse, irregular menstruation, dysmenorrhea, amenorrhea, leukorrhea, pruritis vulvae, frequent urination, and constipation.

Calms the Spirit.
> Indications: night-time epileptic seizures, neurasthenia, and restlessness due to fear.

Moistens the throat.
> Indications: tonsillitis, pharyngitis, sore and dry throat, and dry cough.

Expedites labor.
> Indications: difficult labor and lochioschesis.

K-7 (fù liū)
REPEATED CURRENT

River and Metal point of the Kidney channel.
Located 2 units directly superior to K-3.

Image:
The name refers to this point's function of regulating the body's outflows or currents (sweating, urination, menstruation, etc.).

Functions:
Tonifies the Kidneys (especially Qi, Yang and Yin) and protective Qi, enriches Yin, regulates the Bladder, menstruation and Water Pathways, stimulates or restrains sweating, moistens Dryness, and transforms Damp-Heat.
> Indications: lower Burner-wasting and thirsting syndrome with frequent urination due to Kidney Qi deficiency, malarial disorders, painful urinary dysfunction, acute nephritis, hyperthyroidism with excessive sweating, alternate sensation of heat and cold in the bones, spontaneous or night sweating, common cold, edema, abdominal distention, borborygmus, diarrhea and dysentery, urinary retention and incontinence, dysuria, urethritis, irregular menstruation, and leukorrhea.

Strengthens the back.
> Indications: various types of lower back and kidney pain.

Restores collapsed Yin and unblocks the pulses.
> Indications: heatstroke with excessive sweating, coma and conditions with a collapsed pulse.

Local effect: foot weakness and paralysis.

K-8 (jiāo xìn)
JUNCTION OF FAITHFULNESS

Accumulating point of the Yin-heel vessel on the Kidney channel.

Located 2 units superior to K-3 and 0.5 unit anterior to K-7.

Image:
The name suggests this point's function in promoting faith and confidence, which is vital to maintaining the willpower governed by the Kidneys. It also suggests this point's relationship to and effect on menstruation and the menstrual cycle (likened to the faithful cycles of the ocean tide). The classical meaning of *xin*, heart-felt words which inspire faith, confidence and sincerity, was later included as one of the five virtues (*wu de*). According to some texts, *junction* refers to this point's intersection with the Spleen channel.

Functions:
Tonifies the Kidneys, regulates menstruation, clears Heat, cools Heat in the Blood, and transforms Damp-Heat (especially lower Burner).

Indications: malarial disorders, uterine hemorrhaging, uterine prolapse, urinary retention, dysmenorrhea, irregular menstruation, difficulty bending forward and backward, abdominal pain and swelling, kidney or lower back pain, testicle pain and swelling, night sweats, and diarrhea.

Local effect: inability to flex the foot.

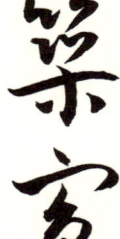

K-9 (zhù bīn)
BUILDING FOR THE GUEST

Accumulating point of the Yin-linking vessel on the Kidney channel.

Located 5 units superior to K-3 on the line connecting K-3 and K-10.

Image:
The name refers to this point's role as an Accumulating point of the Yang-linking vessel on the Kidney channel, which is a building for the guest vessel. Also *bin*, with the bone or flesh radical, means the patella, knee or lower leg. An alternate meaning of *zhu* is "sturdy," which suggests this point's ability to support the patella.

Functions:
Tonifies the Kidneys and regulates the Yin-linking vessel.
    Indications: umbilical hernia in infants, nephritis, cystitis, orchitis, pelvic inflammatory disease, and colic.

Calms the Spirit.
    Indications: insanity, seizures, and depression.

Local effect: pain in the medial aspect of the foot, knee or leg, and gastrocnemius muscle spasm.

K-10 (yīn gǔ)
YIN VALLEY

Sea and Water point of the Kidney channel.

With one knee flexed, located on the medial side of the popliteal fossa level with B-40, between the tendons of the semitendinosus and semimembranosus muscles.

Image:
The name refers to this point's location in a Yin body zone, in a slight depression between two muscles, and its influence on the Yin structures below the umbilicus.

Functions:
Tonifies the Kidneys (especially Yin), clears Heat (especially lower Burner), and Heat in the Blood.

　Indications: hernial disorders, lower abdominal pain, genital pain and itching, impotence, leukorrhea, frequent or painful urination, blood in the urine, uterine bleeding, and diarrhea.

Strengthens the knee.

　Indications: pain, stiffness and swelling in the medial aspect of the knee and thigh.

K-27 (shū fǔ)
CONVEYING PALACE

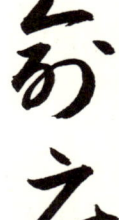

Located 2 units lateral to the Conception vessel in the depression on the lower border of the clavical.

Image:
The name indicates this point's important role in gathering, governing and distributing Qi. *Palace* indicates a place of residence or gathering together, where one commands or rules; *conveying* suggests distribution or transportation. In addition, *fu* (with the flesh radical) refers to the Yang Organs, suggesting the conveyance of Qi from this point to the Yang Organs.

Functions:
Regulates the Lungs, tonifies ancestral Qi, expands and relaxes the chest, and redirects rebellious Qi downward.
> Indications: chronic asthma, bronchitis, stifling sensation in the chest, chest pain, intercostal neuralgia, dyspnea, cough, and headache due to mental strain.

Tonifies the Kidneys (especially Yang), regulates the Stomach, and warms Cold.△
> Indications: generalized sensation of cold, mental fatigue and disorientation, anxiety and palpitations, forgetfulness, nausea, vomiting, lack of appetite, and abdominal distention.

P-1 *(tiān chí)*
HEAVEN'S POOL

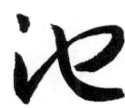

Intersecting point of the Triple Burner, Gallbladder and Liver channels on the Pericardium channel.

Located 1 unit lateral to the nipple in the fourth intercostal space.

Image:
The name refers to the pooling or gathering of the Spirit in the chest region. The Heart and Pericardium govern the Spirit whose symbolic home is heaven. This point's location, its influence on the breast and the storage of milk, is also suggested by the name.

Functions:
Diffuses the Lung Qi, expands and relaxes the chest, regulates Qi, and clears Heat.

> Indications: headache, blurred vision, fever without sweating, cough, dyspnea, stifling sensation in the chest, chest fullness, hypochondriac pain, axillary swelling and pain, fatigued extremities, restlessness, and malaise.

Expedites and facilitates lactation.

> Indications: insufficient lactation and mastitis.

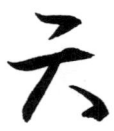

P-2 (tiān quán)
HEAVEN'S SPRING

Located 2 units inferior to the end of the anterior axillary fold between the two heads of the biceps brachii muscle.

Image:
The name refers to this point's classification as a spring or source of pure Qi, originating from the neighboring point P-1 *(tian chi)*, or "Heaven's Pool."

Functions:
Regulates the Heart, expands and relaxes the chest, and invigorates the Blood.
> Indications: stifling sensation, fullness and pain of the chest, distention and pain in the hypochondriac region, pain radiating from the chest to the back, palpitations, and cough.

Local effect: pain radiating down the medial aspect of the upper arm.

P-3 (qū zé)
CURVED MARSH

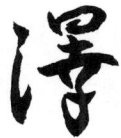

Sea and Water point of the Pericardium channel.

With the elbow flexed, located on the transverse cubital crease at the ulnar side of the tendon of the biceps brachii muscle.

Image:
The name refers to the channel Qi flow at the elbow fold or "curve," where the Qi tends to slow down and spread out before continuing its course.

Functions:
Regulates the Heart (especially Qi) and expands and relaxes the chest.

    Indications: chest fullness, irritability and pain, dyspnea, palpitations, cough, and tremors of the hand and arm.

Regulates the Stomach and Intestines, clears Heat, and cools Heat in the Blood.°

    Indications: heatstroke, urticaria, erysipelas, acute gastroenteritis, fever, excessive thirst, vomiting, stomachache, and diarrhea with blood in the stool.

Local effect: muscular pain and cramps of the arm and elbow.

P-4 (xì mén)
CREVICE GATE

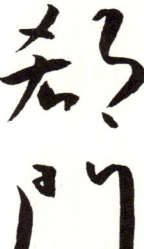

Accumulating point of the Pericardium channel.
Located 5 units proximal to the transverse crease of the wrist on the line connecting P-3 and P-7 between the tendons of the palmaris longus and flexor carpi radialis muscles.

Image:
The name refers to this point's location between two tendons on the wrist. *Crevice* suggests a narrow opening where the Qi and Blood tend to collect. *Xi* is also the term for an Accumulating point.

Functions:
Regulates the Heart (especially Qi).
> Indications: rheumatic heart disease, chest pain, and palpitations.

Calms the Spirit.
> Indications: hysteria, depression, anxiety, palpitations, fear of surroundings and strangers, nervousness, forgetfulness, and insomnia.

Benefits the diaphragm, clears Heat, cools Heat in the Blood, and redirects rebellious Qi downward.
> Indications: chest fullness, irritability and pain due to diaphragm constraint, diaphragmatic spasms, nausea and vomiting, cough or hemoptysis, epistaxis, and boils.

Local effect: pain or paralysis of the anterior forearm and fingers.

P-5 (jiān shǐ)
INTERMEDIARY

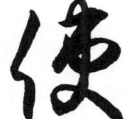

River and Metal point of the Pericardium channel.
Located 3 units proximal to the transverse crease of the wrist on the line connecting P-3 and P-7 between the tendons of the palmaris longus and flexor carpi radialis muscles.

Image:
The name refers to this point's location between two tendons on the wrist. *Intermediary* also suggests this point's influence on the Pericardium, which the classics refer to as the "envoy of the Imperial Heart."

Functions:
Regulates and tonifies the Heart (especially Qi and Yang), expands and relaxes the chest, and transforms Heart Phlegm.
   Indications: rheumatic heart disease, seizures, childhood convulsions, sudden aphasia, chest pain, palpitations, restlessness, excessive salivation due to stroke, and sensation of heat in the palms.

Calms the Spirit.
   Indications: mania, hysteria, depression, hallucinations, insomnia, and aversion to wind and cold.

Clears Heart Fire and Heat, cools Heat in the Blood, and regulates the Stomach.
   Indications: malarial disorders, hyperthyroidism, tidal fever, tonsillitis with fever, scabies, jaundice, stomachache, hemorrhoids, irregular menstruation, and vomiting.

Local effect: pain, stiffness, contracture or twitching of the elbow, forearm or hand.

P-6 (nèi guān)
INNER BORDER GATE

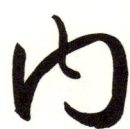
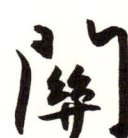

Connecting point of Pericardium channel, Confluent point of the Yin-linking vessel.

Located 2 units proximal to the transverse crease of the wrist on the line connecting P-3 and P-7 between the tendons of the palmaris longus and flexor carpi radialis muscles.

Image:
The name refers to this point's role as the gateway or Connecting point to the Triple Burner channel and the Yin-linking vessel. *Inner* refers to the palmar aspect of the forearm and to the point's location on a Yin channel. This point complements TB-5 *(wai guan)*, the Outer Border Gate.

Functions:
Regulates and tonifies the Heart (especially Qi, Yang, Blood and Yin), transforms Heart Phlegm, facilitates Qi flow, regulates the Yin-linking vessel, and clears Heart Fire.

> Indications: rheumatic heart disease, hyperthyroidism with excessive sweating, chest pain, pain and shock (especially post-surgical), asphyxia due to near drowning, palpitations, and dizziness.

Calms the Spirit and clears the Brain, and dispels Wind-Phlegm.

> Indications: collapsing syndrome, closed-type Wind-stroke, insanity, hysteria, seizures, hyperthyroidism with excessive sweating, stifling sensation in the chest, depression with fullness of the epigastric region, forgetfulness, and insomnia.

Regulates the Liver (especially Qi), Stomach and middle Burner, spreads Liver Qi, clears Fire and Heat, invigorates the Blood, transforms Dampness, Damp-Summerheat and Phlegm, calms the Fetus, and alleviates pain.

> Indications: malarial disorders, dysenteric disorders, restless fetus disorder due to Liver Qi constraint, childhood nutritional impairment with vomiting, acute diseases of the biliary tract, jaundice, pancreatitis, appendicitis, migraine headache, nausea, epigastric pain and distention, hypochondriac pain, diarrhea with vomiting, morning sickness, and irregular menstruation.

Redirects rebellious Qi downward, expands and relaxes the chest, and benefits the diaphragm.

> Indications: asthma, bronchitis, pertussis, hiccups, vomiting, diaphragmatic spasms, intercostal neuralgia, chest fullness and pain, and dyspnea.

Expels gallstones.

Expedites and facilitates lactation.

> Indications: insufficient lactation due to excess, and acute mastitis.

Local effect: contracture and pain in the elbow and arm.

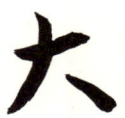
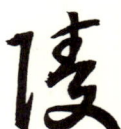

P-7 (dà líng)
BIG MOUND

Source, Stream and Earth point of the Pericardium channel.

At the midpoint of the transverse crease of the wrist, located in the depression between the tendons of the palmaris longus and flexor carpi radialis muscles.

Image:
The name refers to this point's location on the wrist crease at the base of the heel or "mound" of the hand.

Functions:
Regulates the Heart (especially Qi), expands and relaxes the chest and clears Heart Fire.

> Indications: tonsillitis, tongue root pain, palpitations due to fear or fright, intercostal neuralgia, chest and hypochondriac fullness and pain, and swelling of the axilla.

Calms the Spirit and clears the Brain.

> Indications: mania, hysteria with sudden laughing and crying, seizures, insomnia, panic, and fright.

Regulates the Stomach, clears Heat and Summerheat, cools Heat in the Blood.

> Indications: appendicitis, gastritis, scabies, eczema, acne, pimples, conjunctivitis, stomachache, and vomiting.

P-8 *(láo gōng)*
PALACE OF LABOR

Spring and Fire point of the Pericardium channel.

With the palm facing upward, located on the radial side of the third metacarpal bone, proximal to the metacarpophalangeal joint.

Image:
The name suggests manual labor and the point's possible role in physical, mental and spiritual revitalization.

Functions:
Regulates the Heart (especially Qi and Yang), clears Heart Fire, Heat and Summerheat, cools Heat in the Blood, and transforms Damp-Heat.

> Indications: febrile diseases, jaundice, headache, epistaxis, gingivitis, halitosis, thirst, inability to swallow food, chest pain, chest and hypochondriac fullness and pain, excessive sweating of the palms, and fungal infections of the hands and feet.

Revives consciousness and clears the Brain.

> Indications: mania, closed-type Wind-stroke, collapsing syndrome due to excess, stroke, heatstroke, and incoherent speech.

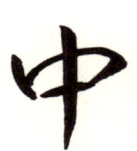
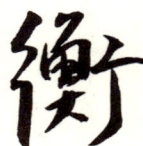

P-9 *(zhōng chōng)*
MIDDLE RUSHING

Well and Wood point of the Pericardium channel.

Located about 0.1 unit from the radial corner of the third fingernail.

Image:
The name refers to this point's location at the terminus of the Pericardium channel and the place where the channel Qi penetrates internally. *Middle* may indicate its location on the third finger as well as its location between the other Yin channels of the arm.

Functions:
Regulates the Heart (especially Qi and Yang), clears Heart Fire, Heat and Summerheat,° benefits the tongue, revives consciousness, and restores collapsed Yang.

> Indications: febrile diseases, childhood convulsions, collapsing syndrome, coma due to Wind-stroke, heatstroke, shock, loss of consciousness, aphasia with stiffening of the tongue, swelling of the underside of the tongue, chest or gastric pain, and sensation of heat in the palms.

TB-1 *(guān chōng)*
GATE'S RUSHING

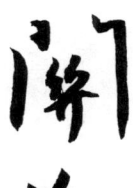
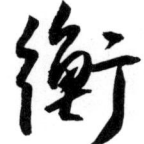

Well and Metal point of the Triple Burner channel.

Located about 0.1 unit from the lateral corner of the fourth fingernail.

Image:
The name refers to this point's location at the beginning of the external channel on the finger, where the vigorous flow of Qi penetrates the barrier or gate to become superficial.

Functions:
Dispels Wind and Wind-Heat, clears Fire and Heat,° revives consciousness, and opens the sensory orifices.

> Indications: malarial disorders, collapsing syndrome, febrile diseases, heatstroke, high fever without sweating, headache, conjunctivitis, blurred vision, deafness, and tinnitus.

Moistens the throat and benefits the tongue.

> Indications: painful obstruction of the throat, tonsillitis, dry mouth, parched lips, and tongue stiffness or flaccidity.

TB-2 (yè mén)
FLUID'S DOOR

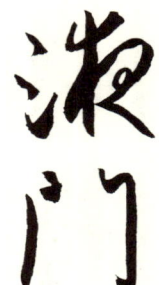

Spring and Water point of the Triple Burner channel.

With the fist slightly clenched, located between the fourth and fifth fingers proximal to the margin of the web.

Image:
The name refers to this point's role in the generation and distribution of Fluids and its classification as a Water point.

Functions:
Clears Heat, dispels Wind, moistens Dryness, and generates Fluids.
> Indications: malarial disorders, febrile diseases, vertigo, headache, conjunctivitis, deafness, tinnitus, gum pain, pain on both sides of the spine, and cold extremities.

Moistens the throat.
> Indications: throat soreness, dryness and swelling, and voice loss.

Local effect: inability of the fingers to extend and flex freely, paralysis of the hand and fingers.

TB-3 *(zhōng zhǔ)*
MIDDLE ISLET

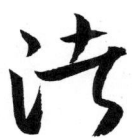

Stream and Wood point of the Triple Burner channel.

With the palm facing downward, located on the back of the hand between the fourth and fifth metacarpal bones in the depression proximal to the metacarpophalangeal joint.

Image:

The name refers to this point's energetic position as the middle point in the classification of the Five Transporting points (Well, Spring, Stream, River and Sea). *Islet* suggests this point's fixed position in the channel's or "river's" course. *Middle* also refers to the Triple Burner's position between the other hand Yang (Large Intestine and Small Intestine) channels.

Functions:

Clears Heat, dispels Wind and Wind-Heat, and moistens Dryness.

> Indications: malarial disorders, fever with sweating, dizziness, headache, intercostal neuralgia, and shoulder pain.

Opens the sensory orifices, moistens the throat, and benefits the ears.

> Indications: various eye disorders including blurred vision and conjunctivitis, deafness, deaf-mutism, tinnitus, otitis media, blocked ears (due to air flight), nasal congestion, throat soreness and dryness, and painful obstruction of the throat.

Local effect: pain and weakness of the fingers, arm and elbow.

TB-4 (yáng chí)
YANG'S POOL

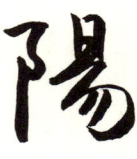
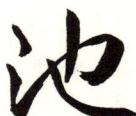

Source point of the Triple Burner channel.

With the palm facing downward, located at the junction of the ulna and carpal bones in the depression lateral to the tendon of the extensor digitorum muscle.

Image:
The name refers to this point's location in a hollow on the mid-dorsal wrist, a Yang body zone. *Pool* or moat suggests an enclosed area of water with raised sides, ideal for gathering Yang Qi.

Functions:
Dispels Wind, clears Fire and Heat, and moistens Dryness.

> Indications: malarial disorders, tonsillitis, common cold, fatigue, tidal fever, painful obstruction of the throat, thirst, dry mouth, chest discomfort, and eye redness and swelling.

Local effect: shoulder, arm and wrist pain.

TB-5 *(wài guān)*
OUTER BORDER GATE

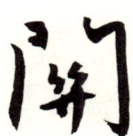

Connecting point of the Triple Burner channel, Confluent point of the Yang-linking vessel.

Located 2 units proximal to TB-4 between the radius and the ulna.

Image:
The name refers to this point's role as a gateway or Connecting point to the Pericardium channel and the Yang-linking vessel. *Outer* refers to the external aspect of the forearm and to its location on a Yang channel. This point complements P-6 *(nei guan)*, the Inner Border Gate.

Functions:
Regulates the Triple Burner and Yang-linking vessel, alleviates exterior conditions, clears Heat, tonifies protective Qi, dispels Wind and Wind-Heat, strengthens and relaxes the sinews, and alleviates pain.

> Indications: febrile diseases, pneumonia, mumps, Wind-predominant painful obstruction, trigeminal neuralgia due to Wind-Heat, upper body atrophy syndrome, hypertension, infantile paralysis, hemiplegia, convulsions, common cold with fever, alternate fever and chills, unilateral or occipital headache, neck stiffness, nausea, vomiting, deafness, tinnitus, chest and hypochondriac pain, shoulder pain and stiffness, severe abdominal pain with cramps, and urinary incontinence.

Local effect: forearm, wrist or finger numbness, contracture or pain, and hand tremor.

TB-6 (zhī gōu)
BRANCH DITCH

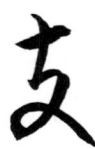
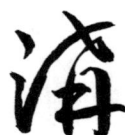

River and Fire point of the Triple Burner channel.
Located 3 units proximal to TB-4 between the radius and the ulna.

Image:
Branch refers to an offshoot, where the linear course of the channel or "ditch" deviates to the next point before resuming its course. *Ditch* may also refer to this point's location between the two bones of the forearm.

Functions:
Regulates the Triple Burner, dispels Wind, Wind-Heat and Wind-Dryness, clears Fire and Heat, transforms Phlegm, moistens Dryness, and generates Fluids.

> Indications: menopausal syndrome, febrile diseases, angina, psoriasis, eczema, pleurisy, edema, lockjaw, tidal fever, vomiting, belching, and shoulder and arm pain.

Expands and relaxes the chest, regulates Qi, facilitates Qi flow and alleviates pain.

> Indications: herpes zoster, chest pain, chest constriction during flu, intercostal neuralgia, axillary, intercostal and hypochondriac pain due to stagnant Qi and Blood, and pain due to cholecystitis.

Regulates and moistens the Large Intestine.

> Indications: fecal incontinence due to paralysis, constipation, and painful defecation.

Expedites lactation.

> Indications: insufficient lactation.

Local effect: pain or motor impairment of the hand and upper extremities.

TB-7 *(huì zōng)*
ASSEMBLY OF THE CLAN

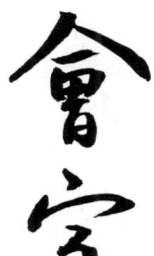

Accumulating point of the Triple Burner channel.

Located 3 units proximal to TB-4 about 0.5 unit lateral to TB-6 on the radial side of the ulna.

Image:
The name suggests a gathering or assembling of the channel Qi at this point and refers to its function as an Accumulating point.

Functions:
Dispels Wind and clears Heat.

> Indications: painful skin conditions, deafness, tinnitus, chest and abdominal fullness and pain, and upper extremity pain and stiffness.

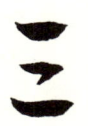
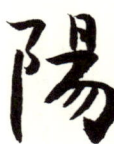
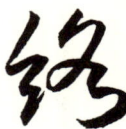

TB-8 *(sān yáng luò)*
THREE YANG CONNECTION

Located 4 units proximal to TB-4 between the radius and the ulna.

Image:
The name refers to the place where the three hand Yang channels approximate each other, suggesting this point's influence on them.

Functions:
Opens the sensory orifices, clears Heat, and dispels Wind.

Indications: upper body atrophy syndrome, deafness, aphasia, sudden mutism or voice loss, lassitude, dizziness and vertigo, severe headache from Wind-Heat, and upper extremity pain and stiffness.

Local effect: pain and motor impairment of the hand and forearm.

TB-10 *(tiān jǐng)*
HEAVEN'S WELL

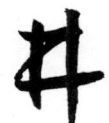

Sea and Earth point of the Triple Burner channel.

With the elbow flexed, in the depression 1 unit superior to the olecranon.

Image:
The name refers to this point's influence on the Spirit and the upper body, both of which correspond to heaven. *Well* suggests a place with a deep and concentrated supply of Qi and refers to this point's position distal to and lower than the "heaven body zone" (the head or skull).

Functions:
Expands and relaxes the chest, redirects rebellious Qi downward, dispels Wind, and clears Heat.

Indications: urticaria, deafness, lack of appetite, tidal fever, excessive sweating, headache, painful obstruction of the throat, cough with purulent sputum or blood, upper body edema, chest and hypochondriac fullness and pain, and pain and swelling in the neck, shoulder or upper arm.

Calms the Spirit and clears the Brain.

Indications: insanity, hysteria, depression, anxiety, and somnolence.

Softens hard masses.

Indications: goiter and scrofula.

Local effect: elbow injuries with pain and stiffness.

TB-14 *(jiān liáo)*
SHOULDER OPENING

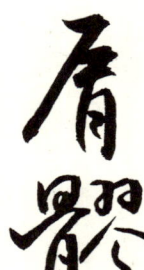

Located on the posterior inferior ridge of the acromion in the depression about 1 unit posterior to LI-15.

Image:
The name refers to this point's location in the depression or opening formed between the posterior-inferior aspect of the acromion and the superior aspect of the head of the humerus.

Functions:
Benefits the shoulders, dispels Wind and Cold,△ and relaxes the sinews.

> Indications: all shoulder conditions including atrophy, inflammation, immobility and pain, urticaria, hypertension, upper-extremity paralysis, and excessive sweating.

TB-17 (yì fēng)
SHIELDING WIND

Intersecting point of the Gallbladder and Triple Burner channels.

Located halfway between the tip of the mastoid process and the angle of the mandible.

Image:
The name refers to this point's function in protecting against and dispelling external pathogenic Wind, especially in the area of the ear and face.

Functions:
Clears the sensory orifices, benefits the ears, dispels Wind and Cold,△ clears Heat, transforms Phlegm, and relaxes the sinews (especially facial).

> Indications: all ear disorders including deafness, tinnitus, otitis media, deaf-mutism and aural vertigo, mania with auditory hallucinations, convulsions, mumps, hypertension, lockjaw, facial paralysis, trigeminal neuralgia, blurred vision, sore eyes, toothache, temporomandibular arthritis or pain, chronic yawning in infants, and sensation of heaviness of the head.

Softens hard masses.

> Indications: scrofula and lymphangitis.

TB-21 (ěr mén)
EAR'S GATE

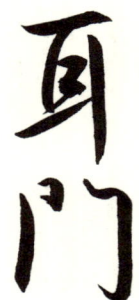

With the mouth slightly open, located in the depression anterior to the supratragic notch and slightly superior to the condyloid process of the mandible.

Image:
The name refers to this point's role as an entry point or gateway of influence to the ear and to its location anterior to the ear canal.

Functions:
Opens and benefits the ears, dispels Wind and Cold,△ and clears Heat.

> Indications: all ear disorders including deafness, tinnitus, otitis media, deaf-mutism, ear abscess and pus in the ear, temporomandibular joint pain or arthritis, headache, and lip stiffness.

TB-23 (sī zhú kōng)
SILKEN BAMBOO HOLE

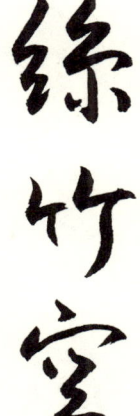

Located in the depression at the lateral corner of the eyebrow.

Image:
The name refers to this point's influence (by way of the lesser connecting channels) on the orbital hollow (shaped like bamboo) which houses the eyes. The lesser connecting channels are also suggested by the image of the small, silky threads that extend into the interior towards the eye. In addition, the eyebrows may be likened to silk or bamboo leaves.

Functions:
Brightens the eyes.
> Indications: all eye disorders including optic nerve atrophy, blurred vision, and color blindness.

Clears Fire and Heat and dispels Wind.
> Indications: seizures, hysteria with vision loss, facial paralysis, conjunctivitis, headache, dizziness, trigeminal neuralgia, and pain in the submandibular region.

Use moxibustion with caution.

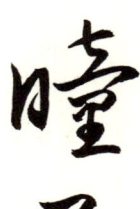
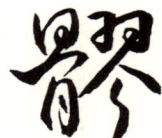

G-1 (tóng zǐ liáo)
PUPIL'S SEAM

Intersecting point of the Small Intestine and Triple Burner channels on the Gallbladder channel.

Located about 0.5 unit lateral to the outer canthus in the depression on the lateral side of the orbit.

Image:
The name refers to this point's location on the bony surface of the outer orbital canthus level with the pupil. *Zi* is the first branch of the twelve earthly branches, corresponding to the time of day (11 P.M.-1 A.M.) associated with the Gallbladder.

Functions:
Brightens the eyes, dispels Wind, and clears Fire and Heat.

    Indications: early-stage glaucomatous disorders, photophobia, conjunctivitis, optic nerve atrophy, night or color blindness, myopia, excessive tearing, trigeminal neuralgia, facial paralysis, and headache.

G-2 (tīng huì)
REUNION OF HEARING

With the mouth open, located in the depression anterior to the intertragic notch directly below SI-19.

Image:
The name expresses this point's strong influence on hearing.

Functions:
Opens and benefits the ears.
> Indications: all ear disorders including deafness, deaf-mutism, tinnitus and otitis media.

Dispels Wind and Cold,△ clears Heat, and relaxes the sinews.
> Indications: convulsions, seizures, hemiplegia, facial paralysis with tinnitus and hearing loss, headache, facial pain, mumps, toothache, and temporomandibular joint pain or arthritis.

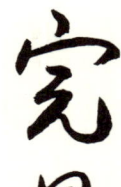
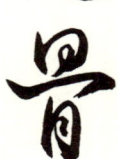

G-12 (wán gǔ)
COMPLETED BONE

Intersecting point of the Bladder channel on the Gallbladder channel.

Located in the depression immediately posterior and inferior to the mastoid process.

Image:
Wan gu is a classical term for the mastoid process, next to which this point is located.

Functions:
Calms the Spirit, dispels Wind and Cold,△ and clears Heat.
> Indications: mania, seizures, aphasia, insomnia, facial swelling or paralysis, headache, dizziness, tinnitus, pain behind the ear, toothache, neck pain and stiffness, and throat pain.

G-14 (yáng bái)
YANG BRIGHTNESS

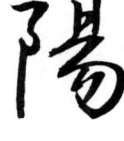
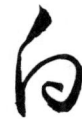

Intersecting point of the Stomach channel and Yang-linking vessel on the Gallbladder channel.

Located directly superior to the pupil, 1 unit above the eyebrow.

Image:
The name suggests this point's function of clearing and brightening the eyes by infusing them with Yang Qi.

Functions:
Brightens the eyes, dispels Wind and Cold,△ and clears Heat.
   Indications: facial paralysis, frontal headache, dizziness, eyelid twitch, conjunctivitis, blurred vision, night blindness, sore eyes, and outer canthus pain.

G-20 (fēng chí)
WIND POOL

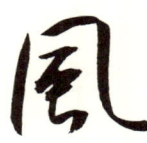
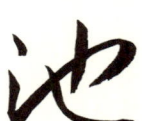

Intersecting point of the Triple Burner channel and the Yang-linking vessel on the Gallbladder channel.

Located below the occipital bones level with GV-16, in the depression between the trapezius and sternocleidomastoid muscles.

Image:
The name refers to the place where external pathogenic Wind easily enters and gathers before penetrating deeper. *Pool* also refers to this point's location in the depression between the trapezius and sternocleidomastoid muscles.

Functions:
Releases exterior conditions, dispels Wind, Wind-Cold,$^\triangle$ Wind-Heat and Cold,$^\triangle$ subdues Liver Yang, relaxes the sinews, facilitates Qi flow, extinguishes Liver Wind, and clears Liver Fire and Heat.

> Indications: malarial disorders, febrile diseases, seizures, muscular tetany, hyperthyroidism with flushed face, hypertension due to Yang excess, painful obstruction with generalized body aches, common cold, urticaria, upper body erysipelas due to Wind-Heat, hemiplegia, insomnia, dizziness and vertigo due to Liver Yang excess, occipital headache, tidal fever, sensation of heaviness of the head, pain and stiffness of the neck and shoulder, lockjaw, neurasthenia due to Liver Yang excess, trigeminal neuralgia, and back pain.

Opens and brightens the eyes.

> Indications: all eye disorders including glaucomatous disorders, optic nerve atrophy, myopia, conjunctivitis, eye soreness and redness, blurred vision, excessive tearing, color, night or sudden blindness, inner canthus redness, and strabismus.

Clears the sensory orifices.

> Indications: closed-type Wind-stroke, painful obstruction of the throat, deafness, tinnitus, sinusitis, and epistaxis.

G-21 (jiān jǐng)
SHOULDER WELL

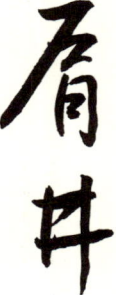

Intersecting point of the Triple Burner channel and Yang-linking vessel on the Gallbladder channel.

Located at the highest point of the shoulder halfway between GV-14 and the acromion.

Image:
The name refers to the deep, concentrated channel Qi at this point, which has a profound effect on shoulder tissue.

Functions:
Spreads Liver Qi, extinguishes Liver Wind, benefits the shoulder, clears Heat, redirects rebellious Qi downward, dispels Wind and Cold,^△ and facilitates Qi flow.

>Indications: aphasia due to Wind-stroke, hemiplegia, vertigo, boils, carbuncles, breast abscess, vertex headache, cough, neck stiffness, chest pain with fever, difficult breathing with profuse mucus, shoulder and back pain, and arm and hand motor impairment.

Expedites labor.
>Indications: lochioschesis and difficult labor.

Facilitates lactation.
>Indications: insufficient lactation and mastitis.

Softens hard masses.
>Indications: scrofula.

Needle with caution during pregnancy or with heart problems.

G-24 (rì yuè)
SUN AND MOON

Alarm point of the Gallbladder.

Located on the mammillary line in the seventh intercostal space.

Image:
The name refers to the expression "clear as the sun and moon," which indicates a person with a quick and decisive mind, a character trait the classical texts associate with the Gallbladder. This point is also associated with the eyes, the sensory orifice influenced by the wood phase Organs. The left eye corresponds to the sun; the right eye corresponds to the moon.

Functions:
Regulates the Liver (especially Qi), Gallbladder and Stomach, redirects rebellious Qi downward, spreads Liver Qi, and transforms Damp-Heat.

Indications: acute diseases of the biliary tract, jaundice, gastric and duodenal ulcers, hypochondriac, intercostal or shoulder pain, intercostal neuralgia, vomiting, acid regurgitation, hiccups, difficulty in speaking, sighing, and fatigued extremities.

Expels gallstones.

G-25 (jīng mén)
CAPITAL GATE

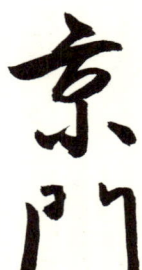

Alarm point of the Kidneys.

Located at the tip of the free end of the twelfth rib.

Image:
The name refers to an entrance or gateway to the "capital" or Kidneys, which house the source Qi and Essence.

Functions:
Tonifies the Kidneys (especially Yang and Yin), regulates the Water Pathways, resolves Dampness, warms the Yang,△ relaxes the sinews, and calms the Fetus.

> Indications: lower Burner-wasting and thirsting syndrome, restless fetus disorder due to Kidney deficiency, painful urinary dysfunction, nephritis, alternate fever and chills, dyspnea, intercostal neuralgia, hypochondriac, abdominal or lower back pain, lower abdominal cramps, kidney pain or prolapse, borborygmus, and diarrhea.

Expels (urinary tract) stones.

> Indications: upper urinary tract stones.

G-26 (dài mài)
GIRDLE VESSEL

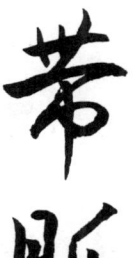

Intersecting point of the Girdle vessel on the Gallbladder channel.

Located directly inferior to Liv-13 at the tip of the free end of the eleventh rib, level with the umbilicus.

Image:
The name indicates this point's influence on the miscellaneous vessel of the same name.

Functions:
Regulates the Girdle vessel and menstruation and transforms Damp-Heat (especially lower Burner).

Indications: hernial disorders, traumatic paraplegia, endometriosis, cystitis, irregular menstruation, leukorrhea due to Damp-Heat, lower abdominal, hip or lower back pain, false urge to urinate or defecate, and diarrhea.

G-27 (wǔ shū)
FIVE PIVOTS

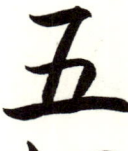

Intersecting point of the Girdle vessel on the Gallbladder channel.

Located 0.5 unit medial to the anterior superior iliac spine and 3 units below the umbilicus, level with CV-4.

Image:
The name refers to this point's function of regulating the Girdle vessel, which crosses five channels on the abdomen: the Kidney, Stomach, Spleen and Liver channels, and the Conception vessel.

Functions:
Regulates menstruation and transforms Damp-Heat (especially lower Burner).

> Indications: hernial disorders, childhood convulsions, colic, endometriosis, irregular menstruation, uterovaginal spasms, leukorrhea, orchitis, retracted scrotum, lower back pain, and lower abdominal pain and distention.

G-28 (wéi dào)
PRESERVING PATH

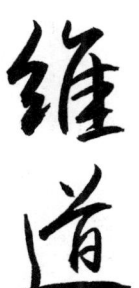

Intersecting point of the Girdle vessel on the Gallbladder channel.

Located 0.5 unit inferior and slightly medial to G-27.

Image:
The name refers to this point's function of preserving the Qi of the Girdle vessel, which binds the abdominal channels together.

Functions:
Moistens and regulates the Intestines and transforms Damp-Heat.
> Indications: colitis, ascites, edema, endometriosis, leukorrhea, irregular menstruation, lower abdominal and lower back pain, and chronic constipation.

Raises middle Qi.
> Indications: uterovaginal prolapse or spasms, intestinal and abdominal hernia.

G-29 (jū liáo)
INHABITED JOINT

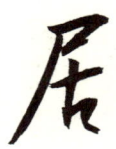
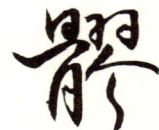

Intersecting point of the Yang-heel vessel on the Gallbladder channel.

Located halfway between the anterior superior iliac spine and the greater trochanter of the femur.

Image:
The name refers to this point's area of influence and location at the head of the femur in the bone socket (the acetabulum).

Functions:
Strengthens the lower back, benefits the hips, relaxes the sinews, dispels Wind and Cold,△ transforms Dampness, and clears Heat.

> Indications: all hip joint disorders, hernial disorders, hemiplegia, lower abdominal and lower back pain, and orchitis.

G-30 *(huán tiào)*
LEAPING CIRCUMFLEXUS

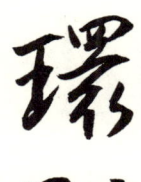
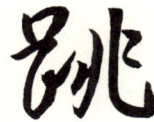

Intersecting point of the Bladder channel and the Gallbladder channel.

Located one-third the distance between the greater trochanter of the femur and the sacral hiatus.

Image:
The name refers to this point's position near the hip joint, a pivot for the circumflexure of the lower extremity, as well as its influence on hip joint mobility. *Leaping*, which suggests rapid movement, refers to the stance a person assumes prior to leaping (legs bent), which aids in the location of this point.

Functions:
Strengthens the lower back, benefits the hips, dispels Wind and Cold,△ clears Heat, strengthens and relaxes the sinews, and transforms Dampness.

> Indications: neurasthenia, urticaria, hemiplegia, edema, lower extremity atrophy syndrome, painful obstruction of the hip and lower extremities, hip joint inflammation, pain and motor impairment of the hip and lower extremities, difficulty in twisting the trunk or straightening the leg, lower back and groin pain, sciatica, and leg Qi.

G-31 (fēng shì)
WIND'S MARKET

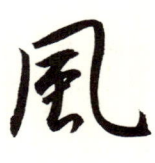

Located on the midline of the lateral aspect of the thigh 7 units superior to the transverse popliteal crease.

Image:
The name refers to this point's location and function as a place for gathering and dispersing pathogenic Wind, especially Wind in the lower extremities.

Functions:
Dispels Wind and Cold,△ clears Heat, relaxes the sinews, and transforms Dampness.

> Indications: urticaria, herpes zoster, hemiplegia, headache, eye redness and swelling, knee and thigh weakness, painful obstruction of the knee and leg, sciatica, leg Qi, lower back pain, and unilateral itching.

G-33 (xī yáng guān)
KNEE YANG HINGE

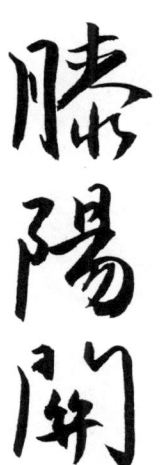

Located approximately 3 units superior to G-34 with the knee flexed, in the depression superior to the lateral epicondyle of the femur and anterior to the tendon of the biceps femoris muscle.

Image:
The name refers to this point's position near the knee, a hinge or strategic barrier for the flow of channel Qi. *Yang* refers to the body zone where this point is found.

Functions:
Strengthens the knee, dispels Wind and Cold,△ transforms Dampness, and clears Heat.

> Indications: rheumatism, generalized pain, knee pain, swelling or immobility, gastrocnemius muscle spasm, and leg Qi.

G-34 (yáng líng quán)
YANG MOUND SPRING

Sea and Earth point of the Gallbladder channel and Influential point of the sinews.
Located in the depression anterior and inferior to the head of the fibula.

Image:
Mound refers to the bony relief of the head of the fibula near this point. *Yang Spring* refers to a deep and pure source of Yang Qi, like a spring at the base of a hill.

Functions:
Regulates and tonifies the Liver (especially Qi, Yang and Blood), regulates the Gallbladder, spreads Liver Qi, subdues Liver Yang, extinguishes Liver Wind, clears Heat, transforms Damp-Heat (especially Liver and Gallbladder) and Damp-Summerheat, and drains Liver pathogens.

> Indications: malarial disorders, hepatitis due to Damp-Heat, Yang-type jaundice, acute biliary tract diseases, lower body erysipelas due to Damp-Heat, cirrhosis of the liver, neurasthenia, headache or hypertension due to Liver Yang excess, head and face swelling, acid regurgitation, painful obstruction of the throat, leg Qi, urinary incontinence, and constipation.

Alleviates exterior conditions, dispels Wind, Wind-Phlegm and Cold,$^\triangle$ benefits the joints and hips, strengthens the knees, strengthens or relaxes the sinews, facilitates Qi flow, regulates Qi, and alleviates pain.

> Indications: Wind-predominant painful obstruction, seizures, convulsions, lower extremity atrophy syndrome, infantile paralysis, muscular tetany, disorders of the muscles and tendons, various hip joint disorders, hemiplegia, hypochondriac and costal fullness and pain, acute lower back pain, knee pain and inflammation, sciatica, and weakness in lateral deviation of the foot.

G-35 *(yáng jiāo)*
YANG'S INTERSECTION

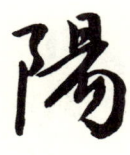

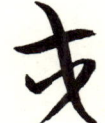

Accumulating point of the Yang-linking vessel.

Located 7 units superior to the vertex of the lateral malleolus on the posterior border of the fibula.

Image:
The name refers to this point's location, where the four foot Yang channels (Gallbladder, Stomach, Bladder and Yang-linking) approximate each other. In addition, the Yang-linking vessel Qi tends to gather at this point.

Functions:
Relaxes the sinews and dispels Wind.
> Indications: asthma, chest and hypochondriac fullness and pain, knee pain and inflammation, gastrocnemius muscle paralysis, and sciatica.

Local effect: pain and cold of the lower leg and foot.

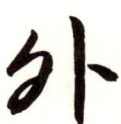

G-36 (wài qiū)
OUTER MOUND

Accumulating point of the Gallbladder channel.

Located 7 units superior to the vertex of the lateral malleolus on the anterior border of the fibula.

Image:
The name refers to the surrounding relief of the fibula and peroneus longus muscle on the lower leg's lateral or outer surface.

Functions:
Regulates the Gallbladder, clears Heat, relaxes the sinews, and resolves Damp-Heat (especially Liver and Gallbladder).

Indications: seizures, hepatitis, muscular tetany, infantile kyphosis, jaundice, headache, neck pain and stiffness, chest and hypochondriac fullness and pain, and abdominal pain.

Local effect: calms muscle spasms.

G-37 *(guāng míng)*
BRIGHT LIGHT

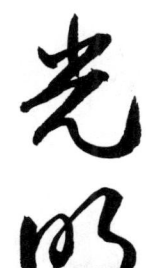

Connecting point of the Gallbladder channel.

Located 5 units superior to the vertex of the lateral malleolus on the anterior border of the fibula.

Image:
The name refers to this point's function of "brightening" and "opening" the eyes.

Functions:
Regulates and tonifies the Liver (especially Yin and Blood) and Gallbladder (especially Qi), dispels Wind, clears Heat, and transforms Damp-Heat.

   Indications: mania, atrophy syndrome or painful obstruction of the lower extremities, fever and chills without sweating, migraine, facial edema, knee pain, and leg Qi.

Opens and brightens the eyes.

   Indications: all eye diseases including optic nerve atrophy, cataract, night or sudden blindness, dim vision, conjunctivitis, eye redness, and pain or itching.

Local effect: pain and spasm of the lower leg and foot.

G-38 (yáng fǔ)
YANG'S ASSISTANT

River and Fire point of the Gallbladder channel.

Located 4 units superior to the vertex of the lateral malleolus on the anterior border of the fibula.

Image:
The name refers to this point's influence on the circulation of Yang Qi and to its location near the fibula. According to the classics, *fu* refers to the fibula, whose role is to assist the tibia.

Functions:
Regulates the Gallbladder, dispels Wind, clears Heat, and transforms Damp-Heat.

> Indications: malarial disorders, hemiplegia, unilateral headache with melancholia, outer canthus pain and redness, bitter taste in the mouth, neck, chest and hypochondriac pain, constipation, knee pain, and generalized aches and pain with stiffness.

Local effect: pain in the lateral aspect of the lower limbs and lower limb paralysis.

G-39 *(xuán zhōng)*
SUSPENDED BELL

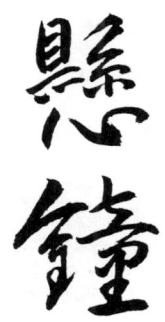

Influential point of the marrow.

Located 3 units superior to the vertex of the lateral malleolus in the depression on the anterior border of the fibula.

Image:
The name refers to a popular custom among children in traditional China of hanging a small bell from the ankle, just above the lateral malleolus (near this point), and suggests this point's ability to affect hearing.

Functions:
Regulates the Gallbladder, extinguishes Liver Wind, dispels Wind, clears Heat, strengthens the bones, and transforms Damp-Heat.

> Indications: Wind-predominant painful obstruction, hemiplegia due to stroke, lower extremity atrophy syndrome, muscular tetany, bone disorders, severe arthritis, lack of appetite, migraine, neck stiffness, abdominal or hypochondriac pain, sciatica, leg Qi, dysuria, painful defecation, and hemorrhoids.

Redirects rebellious Qi downward.

> Indications: painful obstruction of the throat, chest fullness and pain with cough.

Benefits the ears.

> Indications: tinnitus, gradual hearing loss, and deafness.

Local effect: pain and soreness of the lower leg and lateral side of the ankle, weakness in lateral deviation of the foot.

G-40 (qiū xū)
HILL'S RUINS

Source point of the Gallbladder channel.

Located anterior and inferior to the lateral malleolus in the depression on the lateral side of the tendon of the extensor digitorum longus muscle.

Image:
The name, which evokes the image of a collapsed grave or ruin, refers to this point's location in the depression near the external malleolus.

Functions:
Regulates the Liver (especially Qi and Blood) and Gallbladder, spreads Liver Qi, clears Liver Fire and Heat, transforms Damp-Heat (especially Liver and Gallbladder), and benefits the joints.

> Indications: cholecystitis, tidal fever, neck stiffness, vomiting and regurgitation, intercostal neuralgia, dyspnea, lower back, thigh, intercostal and hypochondriac pain, painful obstruction of the lower extremities, and colic.

Softens hard masses.

> Indications: axillary lymphadenitis, scrofula, and goiter.

Local effect: pain, weakness and swelling of the lateral ankle joint.

G-41 *(zú lín qì)*
FOOT VERGE OF TEARS

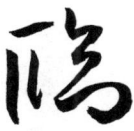

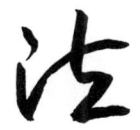

Stream and Wood point of the Gallbladder channel and Confluent point of the Girdle vessel.

Located in the depression distal to the junction of the fourth and fifth metatarsal bones.

Image:
The name refers to this point's ability to promote or halt lacrimation and clear the vision as well as its ability to promote an emotional release through crying.

Functions:
Regulates the Liver (especially Qi), Gallbladder and Girdle vessel, spreads Liver Qi, extinguishes Liver Wind, and transforms Damp-Heat.

   Indications: malarial disorders, irregular menstruation, dysmenorrhea, unilateral or occipital headache, vertigo, chest fullness and pain, dyspnea, intercostal and hypochondriac pain, inflammation of the mastoid process, breast swelling during menstruation, pain and weakness of the lower back and loins, and sciatica.

Brightens the eyes.

   Indications: outer canthus pain and redness, and conjunctivitis.

Softens hard masses.

   Indications: scrofula, axillary and cervical lymphadenitis.

Facilitates lactation.

   Indications: mastitis.

Local effect: pain and swelling of the dorsum of the foot.

G-43 (xiá xī)
BRAVE STREAM

Spring and Water point of the Gallbladder channel.

Located between the fourth and fifth toes proximal to the margin of the web.

Image:
The name refers to the intense channel Qi found at this point. This is evidenced by the strong sensation produced by needling. Its classification also suggests that willpower (a character trait corresponding to the water phase), which bolsters bravery, can be strengthened at this point. Furthurmore, *xia* (with the man radical) means "the space in between," suggesting this point's location in the web between the fourth and fifth toe.

Functions:
Regulates the Gallbladder, clears Heat, subdues Liver Yang, and extinguishes Liver Wind.

> Indications: febrile diseases, hypertension, cerebral congestion, migraine, vertigo, deafness, tinnitus, outer canthus pain and redness, swollen and painful jaw, sore throat, chest and hypochondriac pain, intercostal neuralgia, and anxiety and palpitations.

Local effect: pain and swelling in the dorsum of the foot.

G-44 *(zú qiào yīn)*
FOOT YIN'S APERTURE

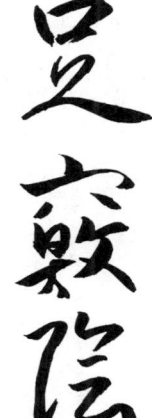

Well and Metal point of the Gallbladder channel.

Located about 0.1 unit from the lateral corner of the fourth toenail.

Image:
The name refers to this point's location at the terminal end or aperture of the Gallbladder channel, where the channel Qi proceeds on to its related Yin (Liver) channel. *Qiao,* which means "orifice," suggests this point's influence on the sensory orifices.

Functions:
Regulates the Gallbladder, subdues Liver Yang, dispels Wind, and clears Heat.
> Indications: febrile diseases, hypertension, dream-disturbed sleep, unilateral headache, vertigo, conjunctivitis, pleurisy, intercostal neuralgia, and dyspnea.

Clears the sensory orifices.
> Indications: blurred vision, eye swelling and redness, deafness, tinnitus, dry mouth, and painful obstruction of the throat.

Local effect: inflammation of the dorsum of the foot.

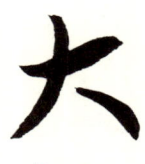

Liv-1 *(dà dūn)*
GREAT SINCERITY

Well and Wood point of the Liver channel.

Located about 0.1 unit from the lateral corner of the first toenail.

Image:
The name refers to this point's position as the first point of the Liver channel, evoking the image of purposeful determination, and perhaps to this point's ability to encourage the expression of this character trait. *Dun* also means "thickness" and suggests the texture of the skin and flesh at this point.

Functions:
Regulates and tonifies the Liver (especially Qi and Blood), spreads Liver Qi, and transforms Damp-Heat (especially lower Burner).

> Indications: genital swelling, pain and inflammation (especially penis and scrotum), penile or scrotal contracture, testicular mumps, urinary tract infection or urinary incontinence, irregular menstruation, unilateral lower abdominal pain, abdominal and inguinal hernia, excessive sweating, and constipation.

Contains the Blood.△

> Indications: all types of bleeding including abnormal uterine bleeding and blood in the urine or stool.

Liv-2 (xíng jiān)
TRAVEL BETWEEN

Spring and Fire point of the Liver channel.

Located between the first and second toe proximal to the margin of the web.

Image:
The name refers to this point's location between the first and second toe at the web along the Liver channel's course, which then proceeds further through the metatarsals.

Functions:
Regulates the Liver (especially Qi and Yang), clears Liver Fire and Heat in the Blood, and invigorates the Blood.

    Indications: hepatitis, jaundice with slight fever, hypertension, neurasthenia, conjunctivitis, dry throat and mouth, diaphragmatic spasms, hypochondriac pain and distention, early menstruation due to Heat in the Blood, menorrhagia, dysmenorrhea, amenorrhea, and abnormal uterine bleeding.

Subdues Liver Yang, extinguishes Liver Wind, and calms the Spirit.

    Indications: seizures, convulsions, mumps, insomnia, headache due to Liver Yang excess, nausea, dizziness and vertigo, tinnitus, intercostal neuralgia, chest fullness and pain, colic, genital pain, and constipation.

Transforms Damp-Heat (especially lower Burner).

    Indications: lower abdominal pain, urinary retention, urinary incontinence, leukorrhea, and diarrhea.

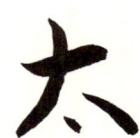
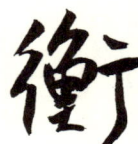

Liv-3 (tài chōng)
GREAT THOROUGHFARE

Source, Stream and Earth point of the Liver channel.

Located in the depression distal to the junction of the first and second metatarsal bones.

Image:
The name refers to this point's function as a strategic and important passageway for the flow of channel Qi. Furthermore, *chong* suggests the intense quality of Qi which can be experienced when needling this point. *Chong* may also allude to the Penetrating vessel, which crosses this point (see *Spiritual Axis*, chapter 38).

Functions:
Regulates and tonifies the Liver (especially Qi, Yang, Blood and Yin), invigorates the Blood, transforms Damp-Heat (especially Liver and Gallbladder), drains Liver Heat, regulates the Gallbladder and menstruation, alleviates pain, and regulates Qi.

> Indications: hepatitis, Yang-type jaundice, hyperthyroidism with flushed face, hernial disorders, menopausal syndrome, early menstruation with profuse bleeding, frigidity, continuous sweating after childbirth, dysuria, urinary incontinence, urinary retention, insomnia,^△ hiccups, shoulder pain, stomachache or epigastric pain due to Liver Qi attack, and lower back pain.

Clears Liver Fire and Heat, cools Heat in the Blood, and redirects rebellious Qi downward.

Indications: glaucomatous disorders, eye pain and redness, trigeminal neuralgia, parietal headache, aural vertigo, nausea and vomiting, morning sickness, sore and dry throat, breast abscess, and constipation with blood in the stool.

Spreads Liver Qi, facilitates Qi and Blood flow, and calms the Fetus.

Indications: collapsing syndrome due to Liver Qi constraint, premenstrual tension due to Liver Qi constraint, restless fetus disorder, irregular menstruation, intercostal neuralgia, and abdominal distention.

Subdues Liver Yang, relaxes the sinews, and extinguishes Liver Wind.

Indications: Wind-predominant painful obstruction, convulsions, muscular tetany, hypertension, dizziness and vertigo due to Liver Yang excess, and temporomandibular joint disorders.

Facilitates lactation.

Indications: insufficient lactation, and mastitis.

Local effect: pain in the medial malleolus and swelling of the dorsum of the foot.

Liv-4 *(zhōng fēng)*
MIDDLE BARRIER

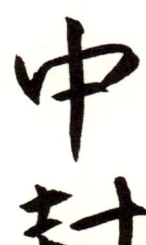

River and Metal point of the Liver channel.

Located on the medial side of the tendon of the tibialis anterior muscles, level with the vertex of the medial malleolus.

Image:
The name suggests a restraining or holding back of the Qi flow at this point, located in the depression on the ankle joint or barrier. *Middle* refers to this point's position on the mid-anterior aspect of the ankle.

Functions:
Regulates the Liver (especially Qi), spreads Liver Qi, clears Heat, and transforms Damp-Heat (especially Liver and Gallbladder).

> Indications: malarial disorders, hernial disorders, jaundice, conjunctivitis, colic, lower abdominal pain and distention, genital pain, seminal emission, and urinary retention.

Local effect: pain and swelling of the ankle joint.

Liv-5 (lí gōu)
DRAINING SHELLS

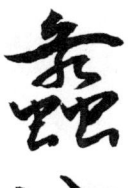
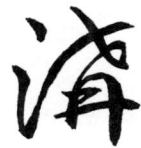

Connecting point of the Liver channel.

Located 5 units superior to the vertex of the medial malleolus on the medial border of the tibia.

Image:
The name signifies purity. The calabash shell (a hollowed-out gourd) was used in Taoist religious and alchemical practice as a sacrificial or measuring vessel due to its Yin-like form and quality. Also, the lateral view of the gastrocnemius muscle is said to resemble a shell. *Draining* refers to this point's classification as a Connecting point.

Functions:
Regulates and tonifies the Liver (especially Yin and Blood), spreads Liver Qi, transforms Damp-Heat (especially lower Burner), stabilizes the Essence,△ enriches Yin, and contains the Blood.△

> Indications: hernial disorders, all types of sexual dysfunction including sterility, impotence, premature ejaculation, involuntary or nocturnal spermatorrhea, orchitis, uterovaginal prolapse, vaginal itching, leukorrhea with or without blood, irregular menstruation, endometriosis and abnormal uterine bleeding, muscle spasms of the back, lower abdominal fullness, urinary retention, and depression.

Liv-6 (zhōng dū)
CENTRAL CAPITAL

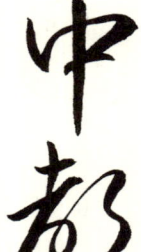

Accumulating point of the Liver channel.

Located 7 units superior to the vertex of the medial malleolus on the medial border of the tibia.

Image:
Capital refers to this point's role as an Accumulating point; *central* refers to its location approximately halfway up the medial aspect of the leg.

Functions:
Spreads Liver Qi and transforms Damp-Heat.
> Indications: hepatitis, hernial disorders, jaundice, hypochondriac or lower abdominal fullness and pain, leukorrhea, and diarrhea.

Liv-8 *(qū quán)*
CURVED SPRING

Sea and Water point of the Liver channel.

With the knee flexed, located in the depression on the medial end of transverse popliteal crease between the upper border of the medial epicondyle of the femur and the tendon of the semimembranosus muscle.

Image:
The name refers to the knee joint that can be flexed or curved and to the pure source of Qi found at this point.

Functions:
Regulates and tonifies the Liver (especially Qi and Blood), drains Liver Heat, spreads Liver Qi, transforms Damp-Heat (especially Liver and Gallbladder), nourishes Blood Dryness, and tonifies the Blood.

> Indications: hernial disorders, dysenteric disorders, painful urinary dysfunction, urinary tract infection, spermatorrhea, testicular mumps, lower abdominal pain, diarrhea, dizziness, and headache.

Regulates menstruation and moves Blood stasis.

> Indications: infertility, uterovaginal prolapse, amenorrhea or dysmenorrhea due to Blood stasis, irregular menstruation, leukorrhea, abdominal pain after childbirth, impotence, and genital itching or pain.

Strengthens the knee.

> Indications: arthritic pain, stiffness and swelling of the knee and medial aspect of the thigh.

Liv-13 *(zhāng mén)*
ORDER GATE

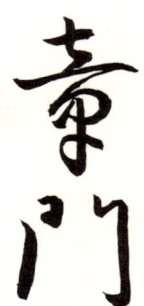

Alarm point of the Spleen, Influential point of the Yin Organs and Intersecting point of the Gallbladder channel on the Liver channel.

Located at the tip of the free end of the eleventh rib.

Image:
The name refers to this point's classification by its ability to influence or create order in the Yin Organs. Also, *zhang*, with the left ear radical, suggests a barrier, and perhaps refers to the rib cage, which protects the internal organs.

Functions:
Regulates, strengthens and tonifies the Spleen (especially Qi and Yang), reduces digestive stagnation, regulates the Stomach and middle Burner, transforms Dampness, Damp-Heat (especially Liver and Gallbladder, Spleen and Stomach) and Phlegm, and warms Cold.△

> Indications: atrophy syndrome due to Damp-Heat, hepatitis, Yin-type jaundice, pancreatitis, ascites, edema, vomiting, indigestion, borborygmus, epigastric pain due to food stagnation, diarrhea due to Cold, and constipation.

Regulates the Liver (Qi, Blood and Yin), spreads Liver Qi, regulates Qi and Blood, and invigorates the Blood.

> Indications: lassitude, intercostal neuralgia, abdominal, hypochondriac and intercostal pain and body tremors, abdominal distention, abdominal masses, and fatigued extremities.

Softens hard masses.

> Indications: enlarged liver and spleen and hard abdominal masses.

Liv-14 (qī mén)
GATE OF HOPE

Alarm point of the Liver, Intersecting point of the Spleen channel and Yin-linking vessel on the Liver channel.

Located on the mammillary line, two ribs below the nipple in the sixth intercostal space.

Image:
The name refers to this point's role in regulating the Liver's command of Qi. When the Liver Qi stagnates, depression can arise, leading to a sense of hopelessness or despair. *Qi* also refers to a complete period or cycle of channel Qi that has passed through all twelve channels at this point. In addition, *qi men* is a classical term for the rank of an army officer (the commander of the royal guards). The *Inner Classic* states that the Liver "functions as a military leader who excels in strategic planning," indicating this point's strong influence on the Liver.

Functions:
Regulates the Liver (especially Qi) and the Gallbladder, spreads Liver Qi, expands and relaxes the chest, and transforms Damp-Heat (especially Liver and Gallbladder).

Indications: malarial disorders, hepatitis, cholecystitis, pancreatitis, hypertension, cirrhosis of the liver, hunger with no desire to eat, acid regurgitation, chest pain, epigastric pain due to Liver Qi constraint, chest and hypochondriac fullness, distention and pain.

Expedites and facilitates lactation.

Indications: insufficient lactation, and mastitis.

CV-1 *(huì yīn)*
MEETING OF YIN

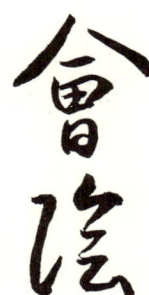

Intersecting point of the Governing and Penetrating vessels on the Conception vessel.

Located at the center of the perineum between the anus and scrotum in males, and between the anus and posterior labial commissure in females.

Image:
The name refers to this point's location on the perineum where the Yin is concentrated. (*Hui yin* is a term for the perineum.) In addition, Yin refers to the reproductive organ outlets and their inferior position on the body. This point also begins the external pathway of the Conception vessel, which regulates the other Yin channels. B-35 *(hui yang)*, or "Meeting of Yang," complements this point.

Functions:
Stabilizes the Essence and the lower orifices, regulates the Conception vessel and menstruation, tonifies and regulates Qi, and clears Heat.

> Indications: hernial disorders, amenorrhea, irregular menstruation, uterovaginal or rectal prolapse, impotence, spermatorrhea, genital or perineal pain, itching and swelling, hemorrhoids, prostatitis, dysuria, urinary retention, night sweats, and constipation.

Calms the Spirit, clears the Brain, and revives consciousness.

> Indications: hysteria, insanity, melancholia, coma, and asphyxia due to near drowning.

CV-2 (qū gǔ)
CROOKED BONE

Intersecting point of the Liver channel on the Conception vessel.

Located just above the pubic symphysis on the anterior midline.

Image:
The name is a classical term for the pubic symphysis.

Functions:
Stabilizes Essence, regulates the Bladder and menstruation, and warms Cold.△

> Indications: impotence, spermatorrhea, orchitis, groin hernia, all urinary problems including uterine inflammation, uterus failing to return to normal shape after childbirth, uterine fibroids and sensation of cold in the uterus, leukorrhea, amenorrhea, dysmenorrhea, and lower abdominal distention and pain.

Raises middle Qi and contains the Blood.△

> Indications: uterine prolapse, hemorrhaging or bleeding.

Use needles or moxibustion with caution during pregnancy.

CV-3 (zhōng jí)
CENTRAL POLE

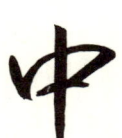
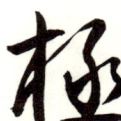

Alarm point of the Bladder, Intersecting point of the Liver, Spleen and Kidney channels on the Conception vessel.
Located 4 units inferior to the umbilicus on the anterior midline.

Image:
The name refers to the pole star around which the other stars revolve, and to this point's location on the abdominal midline or body center. *Central* refers to this point's location at the intersection of three Yin channels on the Conception vessel.

Functions:
Regulates the lower Burner and menstruation, resolves Damp-Heat (especially lower Burner), clears Heat (especially lower Burner), and cools Heat in the Blood.

> Indications: pelvic inflammatory disease, ascites, irregular menstruation, amenorrhea, menorrhagia, uterine fibroids or bleeding, leukorrhea with blood, genital pain or itching, and edema.

Tonifies the Kidneys (especially Qi and Yang), stabilizes Kidney Qi, regulates the Bladder and Water Pathways, and promotes urination.

> Indications: collapsing syndrome, urinary incontinence, retention or infection, dysuria, premature ejaculation, impotence, infertility, prostatitis, lower abdominal pain, and lassitude.

Expels stones (especially urinary tract).

> Indications: lower urinary tract stones.

Use needles or moxibustion with caution during pregnancy.

CV-4 (guān yuán)
HINGE AT THE SOURCE

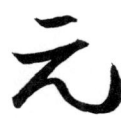

Alarm point of the Small Intestine, Intersecting point of the Liver, Spleen and Kidney channels on the Conception vessel.

Located 3 units inferior to the umbilicus on the anterior midline.

Image:
The name refers to this point's role as a gateway to the source Qi and to its location just within the "cinnabar field" (*dan tian*). *Hinge* refers to a pivotal opening or strategic pass; *source* refers to the source Qi, which this point influences.

Functions:
Tonifies the Kidneys (especially Yang and Yin), tonifies source Qi, regulates the lower Burner and menstruation, tonifies the Qi and Blood,△ warms Cold,△ enriches Yin, and drains pathogenic influences from the Heart.

> Indications: abandoned-type Wind-stroke, seizures, chronic consumptive disorders, lower Burner-wasting and thirsting syndrome with frequent urination, restless fetus disorder due to deficiency, asthma due to Kidney deficiency, pulmonary tuberculosis with chills and shortness of breath, hypertension, neurasthenia, forgetfulness, insomnia, dizziness and vertigo due to Qi and Blood deficiency, emaciation with lassitude, lower abdominal pain, postpartum abdominal pain, lochioschesis, abnormal uterine bleeding, leukorrhea, irregular or prolonged menstruation, and inflamed testicles.

Stabilizes Kidney Qi.

    Indications: syrupy- or Qi-type painful urinary dysfunction, infertility, impotence, spermatorrhea, and headache.

Warms the Yang$^\triangle$ and raises middle Qi.

    Indications: various types of organ prolapse including stomach, rectal and uterine prolapse, abdominal distention and pain, and diarrhea with tenesmus.

Regulates the Small Intestines and the Water Pathways, resolves Dampness and Damp-Heat (especially lower Burner), and dries Dampness$^\triangle$ and Damp-Cold.$^\triangle$

    Indications: dysenteric disorders, chronic nephritis, dysuria, urinary incontinence, chyluria, urinary tract infection, and prostatitis.

Restores collapsed Yang$^\triangle$ or Yin.

    Indications: abandoned-type Wind-stroke, abandoned-type coma, collapsing syndrome with cold extremities, shock, generalized weakness, tidal fever, and thirst.

Use needles or moxibustion with caution during pregnancy.

CV-5 (shí mén)
STONE GATE

Alarm point of the Triple Burner.
Located 2 units inferior to the umbilicus on the anterior midline.

Image:
Shi, which means stone or mineral, refers to cinnabar, the most highly-prized mineral to Taoist alchemists who believed that because of its near-perfect balance of Yin and Yang, and its ability to nourish source Qi (stored in the area between CV-4 and CV-7), the proper preparation and ingestion of this substance could impart immortality. Cinnabar also symbolized the state of open consciousness associated with meditation. *Men*, which means gate, refers to this point's location at the center of the "cinnabar field" (*dan tian*), another name for this point, and a body region which contains the sperm, or the uterus. In ancient times, needling or moxa cauterizing this point was either forbidden or performed with extreme care, because a disruption or dissipation of the source Qi was believed to cause serious side effects including frigidity, impotence, sterility, or a shortened life span. (The expression "stone woman" [*shi nu*] means barren or sterile.)

Functions:
Tonifies the Kidneys (especially Yang), tonifies source Qi, regulates menstruation and the lower Burner, warms the Yang and warms Cold,$^\triangle$ and dries Dampness$^\triangle$ and Damp-Cold.$^\triangle$

> Indications: hernial disorders, leukorrhea, amenorrhea, postpartum hemorrhage, edema, cold, pain and distention in the abdominal region, urinary incontinence or retention, chronic diarrhea, scrotal contraction with retracted testicles, and lack of appetite.

The classical texts prohibit needling.

CV-6 (qì hǎi)
SEA OF QI

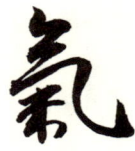

Located 1.5 units inferior to the umbilicus on the anterior midline.

Image:
The name refers to this point's location within and influence on the "cinnabar field" (see CV-5) where the source Qi gathers in a sea-like reservoir.

Functions:
Tonifies the Kidneys (especially Qi and Yang), tonifies source Qi, enriches Yin, regulates the Conception vessel and menstruation, regulates the lower Burner, tonifies the Qi△ and Blood,△ regulates the Water Pathways, resolves Dampness and Damp-Heat, dries Dampness△ and Damp-Cold,△ clears deficiency Heat, cools Heat in the Blood, and calms the Fetus.

> Indications: chronic diarrhea or dysenteric disorders due to Damp-Cold, lower Burner-wasting and thirsting syndrome, restless fetus disorder due to deficiency, menopausal syndrome, asthma due to Kidney deficiency, painful urinary dysfunction, hypertension due to Yang deficiency, neurasthenia, forgetfulness, anxiety and palpitations due to Qi and Blood deficiency, insomnia, stomachache, abdominal masses, irregular menstruation, dysmenorrhea, uterine bleeding, postpartum hemorrhage, lochiaschesis, leukorrhea with blood, periumbilical pain, spermatorrhea, scrotal pain or inflammation, and urinary incontinence.

Restores collapsed Yang△ or Yin, raises middle Qi, warms the Yang,△ and warms Cold.△

Indications: collapsing syndrome due to deficiency, abandoned-type Wind-stroke, abandoned-type coma, heatstroke, Cold-predominant painful obstruction, shock, all types of organ prolapse including uterovaginal, stomach, rectal and intestinal, headache due to Kidney Qi deficiency, epigastric pain due to Stomach deficiency and Cold, generalized body weakness with cold extremities, impotence, and diarrhea due to Kidney Qi deficiency.

Expels stones (especially urinary tract).

Indications: upper urinary tract stones.

CV-7 (yīn jiāo)
YIN JUNCTION

Intersecting point of the Penetrating vessel on the Conception vessel.

Located 1 unit inferior to the umbilicus on the anterior midline.

Image:
The name refers to the Yin energies of the Conception vessel and Penetrating vessel that converge and gather at this point.

Functions:
Tonifies the Kidneys (especially Yang), regulates menstruation and the lower Burner, clears deficiency Heat, cools Heat in the Blood, resolves Dampness and Damp-Heat, dries Dampness,△ and Damp-Cold.△

> Indications: neurasthenia, night sweats, edema, abdominal fullness, sensation of heat or itching below the umbilicus, periumbilical pain, knee and back pain, menstrual cramps, dysmenorrhea, abnormal uterine bleeding, amenorrhea, leukorrhea, vaginal itching or discharge, testicle pain, and anxiety.

Use needling and moxibustion with caution during pregnancy.

CV-8 (shén què)
SPIRIT'S PALACE GATE

Located in the center of the umbilicus.

Image:
The name refers to the place where the life force or Spirit enters during fetal development. *Palace Gate* suggests entry and protection. *Shen que* is a modern term for the umbilicus.

Functions:
Tonifies, strengthens and regulates the Spleen (especially Qi and Yang)△ and Stomach (especially Qi),△ regulates the Intestines,△ warms the interior,△ and reduces digestive stagnation.△

> Indications: various gastrointestinal disorders due to deficiency or Cold, headache due to deficiency, lip swelling, abdominal pain and cold, periumbilical pain, and acute or chronic diarrhea due to deficiency or Cold.

Tonifies the Kidneys (especially Yang),△ warms the Yang,△ regulates the Water Pathways,△ restores collapsed Yang,△ and dries Dampness△ and Damp-Cold.△

> Indications: all urinary disorders including painful urinary dysfunction, urinary incontinence and retention, abandoned-type Wind-stroke, restless fetus disorder, collapsing syndrome with chills and cold extremities, heatstroke, shock, neurasthenia, edema, abdominal pain, rectal prolapse due to deficiency, and leukorrhea with blood.

Needling is contraindicated.

CV-9 *(shuǐ fēn)*
WATER DIVIDE

Located 1 unit superior to the umbilicus on the anterior midline.

Image:
The name refers to this point's ability to regulate the Water Pathways, including the Small Intestine's function of separating the pure from the impure. According to classical sources, this point is located directly above the Small Intestine.

Functions:
Regulates the Spleen, Stomach and Small Intestine, warms Cold,△ regulates the Water Pathways, and resolves Dampness.

> Indications: nephritis, ascites, edema, lack of appetite, borborygmus, abdominal pain, coldness and swelling, periumbilical pain or cold, diarrhea, urinary retention, dysuria, lower back pain, and palpitations.

CV-10 (xià wăn)
LOWER STOMACH CAVITY

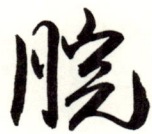

Intersecting point of the Spleen channel on the Conception vessel.

Located 2 units superior to the umbilicus on the anterior midline.

Image:
The name refers to this point's action on the lower part of the stomach cavity and its ability to link and harmonize the middle and lower Burners by way of the Conception vessel.

Functions:
Regulates the Spleen and Stomach (especially Qi), transforms Dampness and Damp-Heat, and reduces digestive stagnation.

> Indications: dysenteric disorders, gastritis, duodenal ulcer, abdominal masses, lack of appetite, epigastric pain and distention, abdominal pain and distention, indigestion, borborygmus, and diarrhea.

CV-11 *(jiàn lǐ)*
BUILD WITHIN

Located 3 units superior to the umbilicus on the anterior midline.

Image:
The name refers to this point's action on the digestive organs (Stomach, Spleen and Small Intestine), whose function it is to build and construct the nutritive Qi. *Jian*, with the man radical, is a medical term meaning to strengthen the Spleen's transporting and transforming function.

Functions:
Regulates and strengthens the Spleen (especially Qi), regulates the Stomach (especially Qi), tonifies nutritive Qi, and transforms Dampness and Damp-Heat.
> Indications: gastritis, ascites, abdominal pain and swelling, edema, stomachache due to food stagnation, lack of appetite, indigestion, and borborygmus.

Redirects rebellious Qi downward.
> Indications: vomiting and chest pain.

CV-12 *(zhōng wǎn)*
MIDDLE STOMACH CAVITY

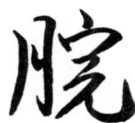

Alarm point of the Stomach, Influential point of the Yang Organs, Intersecting point of the Small Intestine, Triple Burner and Stomach channels on the Conception vessel.

Located 4 units superior to the umbilicus on the anterior midline.

Image:
The name refers to this point's influence on the middle part of the stomach cavity and its ability to harmonize the middle Burner.

Functions:
Regulates, strengthens and tonifies the Spleen (especially Qi and Yang), regulates the Stomach (especially Qi and Yin) and middle Burner, tonifies nutritive Qi, reduces digestive stagnation, regulates Qi and Blood, warms Cold,^△ transforms Dampness, Damp-Heat and Phlegm, dries Damp-Cold,^△ and calms the Fetus.

> Indications: middle Burner-wasting and thirsting syndrome with emaciation, dysenteric disorders due to Damp-Cold, atrophy syndrome due to Damp-Heat, childhood nutritional impairment, restless fetus disorder, pulmonary tuberculosis with suppressed appetite, neurasthenia, fatigue after childbirth, jaundice, acute and chronic gastritis, stomach and duodenal ulcers, indigestion, headache due to indigestion, lack of appetite, stomachache, epigastric pain, abdominal distention and pain, borborygmus, diarrhea, constipation, stool with undigested food, and diarrhea.

Redirects rebellious Qi downward, clears Stomach Fire and Heat.

Indications: morning sickness, vomiting, acid regurgitation, dizziness and vertigo, hiccups, burning sensation in the esophagus and throat, and chest and stomach pain.

Raises middle Qi.

Indications: stomach or other upper abdominal organ prolapse.

CV-13 *(shàng wăn)*
UPPER STOMACH CAVITY

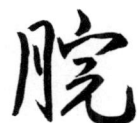

Intersecting point of the Small Intestine and Stomach channels on the Conception vessel.

Located 5 units superior to the umbilicus on the anterior midline.

Image:
The name refers to this point's action on the upper stomach cavity and its ability to link and harmonize the upper and middle Burners by way of the Conception vessel.

Functions:
Regulates the Spleen and Stomach, clears Stomach Fire, transforms Dampness and Damp-Heat, and warms the interior.[△]

> Indications: jaundice, stomach and duodenal ulcers, morning sickness, lack of appetite, excessive salivation, hiccups due to Cold, indigestion, epigastric pain, stomachache, abdominal distention, and diarrhea.

Regulates the Heart (especially Qi) and calms the Spirit.

> Indications: seizures, insanity, incoherent speech, palpitations, chest pain, anxiety, and fear.

Redirects rebellious Qi downward.

> Indications: vomiting and cough with sputum.

CV-14 (jù què)
GREAT PALACE GATE

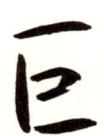
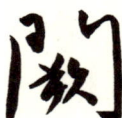

Alarm point of the Heart.

Located 6 units superior to the umbilicus on the anterior midline.

Image:
The name suggests entrance and protection. *Palace* refers to the "home of the emperor" or the Heart. Also, *ju que* is a term for a sword from ancient times which the xiphoid and sternum were thought to resemble.

Functions:
Regulates the Heart (especially Qi), transforms Heart Phlegm, calms the Spirit, and regulates the Qi.
> Indications: collapsing syndrome with chills, forgetfulness, lassitude, chest pain, stifling sensation in the chest, palpitations due to fear, and cold extremities.

Benefits the diaphragm, regulates the Stomach, transforms Phlegm, and redirects rebellious Qi downward.
> Indications: jaundice, vomiting, regurgitation, hiccups, difficulty in swallowing, diaphragmatic spasms, shortness of breath, stomachache, upper abdominal distention, cold extremities, and diarrhea.

Calms the Spirit.
> Indications: insanity, hysteria, depression, fear, and anxiety.

CV-15 *(jiū wěi)*
TURTLEDOVE TAIL

Connecting point of the Conception vessel.

Located 7 units superior to the umbilicus on the anterior midline.

Image:
The name is a classical term for the xiphoid process. The sternum is thought to resemble a bird, the ribs being the wings.

Functions:
Regulates the Heart, expands and relaxes the chest, calms the Spirit, and transforms Heart Phlegm.

> Indications: hysteria, mania, pericarditis, chest pain, palpitations, and fear and fright.

Redirects rebellious Qi downward, dispels Wind, clears Heat, and benefits the diaphragm.

> Indications: seizures, asthma, lassitude, mental exhaustion, vomiting, acid regurgitation, cough, sore throat, hiccups, diaphragmatic spasms, stomachache, and abdominal migraine.

CV-17 (tán zhōng)
CENTRAL ALTAR

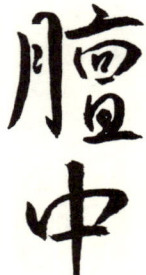

Alarm point of the Pericardium, Influential point of the Qi and Sea of Qi point.

Located between the nipples, level with the fourth intercostal space on the anterior midline.

Image:
The name refers to this point's location at the center of the chest, seated on an "altar" (the sternum) or "place of worship" where the Spirit resides. The classical term for the exposed middle portion of the chest was *tan zhong*, which today means the sternum.

Functions:
Regulates the Lungs (especially Qi) and the upper Burner, tonifies ancestral Qi, expands and relaxes the chest, diffuses Lung Qi, regulates and tonifies Qi, transforms Phlegm (especially chest), Phlegm-Cold$^\triangle$ and Phlegm-Heat, and warms the Yang.$^\triangle$

> Indications: pulmonary tuberculosis with shortness of breath, bronchitis, asthma, Lung Abscess, menopausal syndrome, inability to speak due to deficiency, labored breathing, facial pallor, chest pain, palpitations, intercostal neuralgia, hypochondriac constriction and pain, diaphragmatic spasms, and anxiety.

Redirects rebellious Qi downward.

> Indications: stifling sensation in the chest, hiccups, coughing of blood or sputum, and difficulty or inability to swallow food with esophageal dryness.

Facilitates and expedites lactation.

> Indications: all breast disorders including acute mastitis, insufficient lactation and breast abscess.

CV-22 *(tiān tū)*
HEAVEN'S CHIMNEY

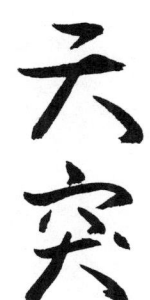

Intersecting point of the Yin-linking vessel on the Conception vessel.

Located in the depression on the suprasternal fossa on the anterior midline.

Image:
The name refers to the throat, especially the trachea, which protrudes upward toward heaven (the head and skull) by way of the neck.

Functions:
Regulates the Lungs (especially Qi), diffuses Lung Qi, and transforms Phlegm.

> Indications: acute and chronic asthma, bronchitis, Lung Abscess, common cold with sore and swollen throat, lung and throat mucus, and chest pain radiating to the back with labored breathing.

Moistens the throat, softens hard masses, and redirects rebellious Qi downward.

> Indications: hysteria with voice loss or hiccups, voice loss, esophageal spasms, throat pain, dryness or swelling with inability to swallow food, vomiting, hiccups, coughing of blood or sputum, and tongue stiffness.

Deep needling is contraindicated.

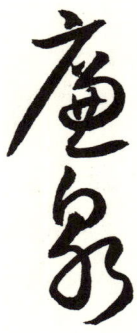

CV-23 *(lián quán)*
PURE SPRING

Intersecting point of the Yin-linking vessel on the Conception vessel.

Superior to the laryngeal prominence, located at the superior ridge of the hyoid bone on the anterior midline.

Image:
The name refers to the quality of Qi and the influence of this point on the salivary glands.

Functions:
Moistens the throat, benefits the tongue, clears Fire and Heat, transforms Phlegm, and generates Fluids.

> Indications: wasting and thirsting syndrome with intense thirst, closed-type Wind-stroke with aphasia and tongue stiffness, swelling or pain, hysteria with voice loss, asthma, tonsillitis, pharyngitis, deaf-mutism, mouth and tongue ulcers, tongue paralysis or stiffness, sudden aphasia, sudden voice loss, spasm of the larynx, hypersalivation, dry tongue and mouth, cough, and catarrh.

Use moxibustion with caution.

CV-24 (chéng jiāng)
RECEIVING LIQUID

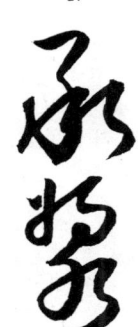

Intersecting point of the Stomach and Large Intestine channels and Governing vessel on the Conception vessel.

Located in the depression inferior to the mentolabial groove on the anterior midline.

Image:
The name refers to this point's location on the chin in the depression below the middle of the lower lip where saliva and thick liquids accumulate. *Cheng jiang* is a term for the mentolabial sulcus.

Functions:
Dispels Wind and Cold,△ clears Heat, transforms Dampness and Phlegm, and relaxes the sinews (especially facial).

Indications: seizures, lockjaw, hemiplegia, facial paralysis, facial swelling, sudden voice loss, excessive salivation, excessive thirst, mouth and tongue ulcers, gingivitis, gum or tooth pain, lip tension, and melancholia.

GV-1 (cháng qiáng)
LASTING STRENGTH

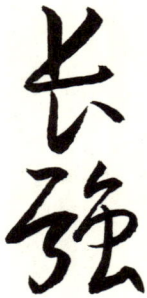

Connecting point of the Governing vessel, Intersecting point of the Gallbladder and Kidney channels on the Governing vessel.

Located midway between the coccyx and anus.

Image:
The name refers to this point's role in giving strength and vitality to the whole spinal column and the Governing vessel.

Functions:
Regulates the Governing vessel and calms the Spirit.
> Indications: hysteria, insanity, seizures, convulsions, muscular tetany, depression, fatigue and lassitude, scrotal eczema or pain, and spermatorrhea due to fright.

Regulates the Intestines, clears Heat, cools Heat in the Blood, and stabilizes the lower orifices.
> Indications: rectal prolapse, hemorrhoids, blood in the stool, diarrhea, constipation, and fecal incontinence.

Strengthens the lower back.
> Indications: lower back and sacral pain, spinal stiffness, and muscular cramps.

GV-2 *(yāo shū)*
LUMBAR'S HOLLOW

Located in the sacral hiatus on the posterior midline.

Image:
The name refers to this point's relationship with and influence on the waist and lumbosacral area. *Hollow* suggests a container or conveyor through which the circulating Qi passes (see B-13 [*fei shu*]).

Functions:
Strengthens the lower back and dispels Wind and Cold.△

  Indications: seizures, lower extremity atrophy syndrome, amenorrhea, lower back or sacral pain, chills and stiffness, urinary incontinence, and hemorrhoids.

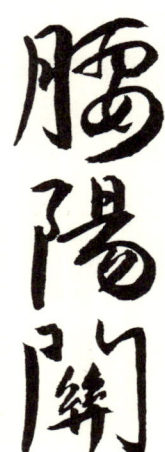

GV-3 *(yāo yáng guān)*
LUMBAR YANG'S HINGE

Located inferior to the spinous process of the fourth lumbar vertebra on the posterior midline.

Image:
The name refers to this point's location at the junction or border of Yin and Yang (Yin corresponds to the lower body; Yang to the upper body). This point regulates Yin and Yang and acts as an important joint or hinge that influences lower back mobility.

Functions:
Tonifies the Kidneys (especially Qi and Yang), stabilizes Kidney Qi, benefits the lower back and knees, warms Cold,△ and dries Damp-Cold.△

> Indications: nephritis, colitis, irregular menstruation, leukorrhea, impotence, premature ejaculation, lumbar disc problems, lower back pain, lower abdominal distention, knee pain or weakness, leg cramps or paralysis, and diarrhea due to Damp-Cold.

GV-4 (mìng mén)
VITAL GATE

Located inferior to the spinous process of the second lumbar vertebra on the posterior midline.

Image:
The name refers to this point's important role in nourishing and stabilizing the Kidneys and "cinnabar field" (see CV-5). In Taoism, the area on the back level with the umbilicus to about 3 units below is considered a corridor for the source Qi, Kidney Qi and Essence which, depending on their relative strength or weakness, make up the body's basal vitality level.

Functions:
Tonifies the Kidneys (especially Qi and Yang), tonifies source Qi, regulates the Water Pathways, dries Dampness and Damp-Cold,$^\triangle$ warms the Yang$^\triangle$ and warms Cold,$^\triangle$ and benefits the lower back and bones.$^\triangle$

> Indications: bone disorders, chronic nephritis, myelitis, neurasthenia due to Kidney Yang deficiency, irregular menstruation, amenorrhea, leukorrhea, abnormal uterine bleeding due to Kidney Yang deficiency, lower back stiffness and pain, kidney pain radiating to the abdomen, hemorrhoids, urinary incontinence, dysuria, blood in the stool due to Cold, and diarrhea.

Tonifies Essence,$^\triangle$ stabilizes Kidney Qi,$^\triangle$ and calms the Fetus.

> Indications: atrophy syndrome due to Essence deficiency, restless fetus disorder due to Kidney deficiency, and all sexual dysfunctions including impotence and sterility.

Calms the Spirit, benefits and clears the Brain, and restores collapsed Yang.△

Indications: seizures, mania, childhood convulsions, meningitis, anemia, disorientation due to deficiency, forgetfulness, fear and fright, insomnia, somnolence, dizziness, tinnitus, and cold extremities.

GV-5 *(xuán shū)*
SUSPENDED AXIS

Located inferior to the spinous process of the first lumbar vertebrae on the posterior midline.

Image:
The name refers to the channel Qi which is in transition at this point (situated between the lower and middle Burners). It also refers to the general area surrounding this point, which resembles a suspended axis or pivot for lumbar movement when a person assumes the supine position.

Functions:
Regulates and tonifies the Spleen (especially Qi and Yang), regulates the Stomach, and benefits the lower back.

> Indications: abdominal pain and distention, indigestion, lower back pain and stiffness, diarrhea with undigested food, and hemorrhoids.

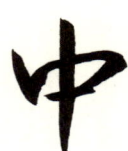
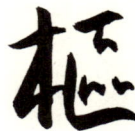

GV-7 *(zhōng shū)*
CENTRAL AXIS

Located inferior to the spinous process of the tenth thoracic vertebrae on the posterior midline.

Image:
The name refers to this point's location within and influence on the middle Burner.

Functions:
Regulates the Spleen and Stomach and benefits the back.
> Indications: cholecystitis, spinal stiffness and pain, epigastric, abdominal or mid-back pain, stomachache, and indigestion.

GV-9 (zhì yáng)
SUPREME YANG

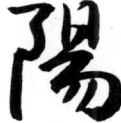

Located inferior to the spinous process of the seventh thoracic vertebra on the posterior midline.

Image:
The name suggests an overabundance of Yang Qi, which is dispersed and redistributed at this point. In addition, it refers to this point's location on the Governing vessel, the back, and at the seventh thoracic vertebra, all of which correspond to Yang.

Functions:
Regulates the Liver and Gallbladder, strengthens the back, spreads Liver Qi, clears Liver Fire and Heat, and transforms Damp-Heat (especially Liver and Gallbladder).

Indications: malarial disorders, hepatitis, jaundice, cholecystitis, bronchiectasis, asthma and cough, chest pain, distending pain in the hypochondrium, lack of appetite, abdominal pain and distention, cold sensation in the stomach, borborygmus, and extremity edema.

Local effect: spinal stiffness and pain.

GV-10 (líng tái)
SPIRIT'S PLATFORM

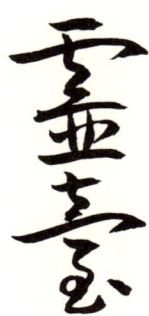

Located inferior to the spinous process of the sixth thoracic vertebra on the posterior midline.

Image:
The name refers to this point's position on a platform one vertebra below the place where the Spirit emanates from the Heart and its related points (GV-11, B-15 and B-44).

Functions:
Expands and relaxes the chest, strengthens the back, and clears Heat.

> Indications: malarial disorders, asthma, bronchitis, cough, neck pain and stiffness, upper back pain, and boils.

GV-11 *(shén dào)*
SPIRIT'S PATH

Located inferior to the spinous process of the fifth thoracic vertebra on the posterior midline.

Image:
The name refers to this point's close relationship with B-15 *(xin shu)*, or "Heart's Hollow," and B-44 *(shen tang)*, or "Spirit's Hall," points that reflect the Spirit or its lodging place, the Heart. *Path* suggests a connection or entrance.

Functions:
Regulates the Heart (especially Qi and Yang), expands and relaxes the chest, calms the Spirit, and dispels Wind.

Indications: asthma, cough, chest and hypochondriac pain, anxiety and palpitations due to fear, neurasthenia, aphasia due to Wind-stroke, forgetfulness, and insomnia.

GV-12 *(shēn zhù)*
BODY'S PILLAR

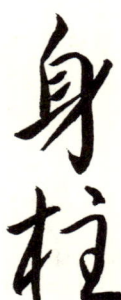

Located inferior to the spinous process of the third thoracic vertebra on the posterior midline.

Image:
The name refers to this point's role in holding up the neck and head from its position in the upper thoracic vertebrae, and to its assistance in strengthening the back.

Functions:
Regulates the Lungs (especially Qi), diffuses Lung Qi, expands and relaxes the chest, calms the Spirit, dispels Wind and Wind-Heat, and clears Heat.

> Indications: insanity, hysteria, febrile convulsions, tuberculosis, asthma, bronchitis, bronchiectasis, pertussis, cough, lower back pain and stiffness, neurasthenia, headache and fever, fever due to excess, neck and upper back stiffness and pain, and boils.

GV-13 (táo dào)
MOULDED PATH

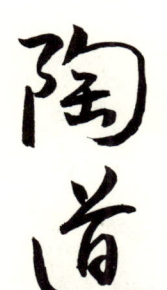

Intersecting point of the Bladder channel on the Governing vessel.

Located inferior to the spinous process of the first thoracic vertebra on the posterior midline.

Image:
Moulded refers to the ceramic and earthenware amulets used by the Taoists to ward off evil spirits believed responsible for fevers and other disorders. *Moulded* can also mean nurtured, uplifted or cultivated. Both interpretations suggest this point's function in strengthening the protective Qi and nurturing the Spirit.

Functions:
Tonifies protective Qi, diffuses Lung Qi, calms the Spirit, clears Fire and Heat, dispels Wind and Wind-Heat, and relaxes the sinews.

> Indications: febrile diseases, malarial disorders, tuberculosis, mania, steaming bone syndrome, muscular tetany, asthma, tidal fever, fever and chills, neck, shoulder, upper back and spine stiffness, pain and cramps, headache due to neck stiffness, insomnia, cough, and chest pain.

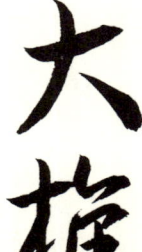

GV-14 (dà zhuī)
BIG VERTEBRA

Influential point of the Yang, Sea of Qi point.

Located inferior to the spinous process of the seventh cervical vertebra on the posterior midline.

Image:
The name refers to this point's location below the prominent seventh vertebra.

Functions:
Calms the Spirit and clears the Brain.
> Indications: mania, melancholia, headache, hysteria, difficulty in breathing deeply and difficulty in speaking.

Tonifies protective Qi, reduces fever, facilitates Qi flow, regulates Qi, dispels Wind and Wind-Heat, clears Fire, Heat and Summerheat, restores collapsed Yin, and relaxes the sinews.
> Indications: all febrile diseases, malarial disorders, steaming bone syndrome, febrile convulsions, seizures, atrophy syndrome due to Lung Heat, closed-type coma, pulmonary tuberculosis, emphysema, hepatitis, urticaria and eczema due to Wind-Heat, Wind-predominant painful obstruction with fever, heatstroke, muscular tetany, hemiplegia, hypertension, common cold due to Wind-Heat, sensation of fullness in the chest, tidal fever, fever and chills, pertussis, spinal stiffness, and neck stiffness and pain.

GV-15 (yǎ mén)
GATE OF MUTENESS

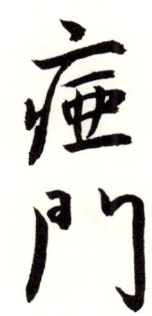

Sea of Qi point.

Located 0.5 unit inferior to GV-16 on the posterior midline between the first and second cervical vertebrae.

Image:
The name reveals this point's action on the voice and related physical structures.

Functions:
Clears the Brain, benefits the tongue, moistens the throat, and facilitates Qi flow.

> Indications: closed-type Wind-stroke with aphasia and tongue stiffness, seizures, mania, hysteria, developmental disorders, mumps, seizures, sudden aphasia, tongue stiffness, swelling or paralysis, tinnitus, deaf-mutism, congenital deafness, cerebral congestion, headache, sensation of heaviness of the head, throat swelling, and neck pain and stiffness.

Deep needling is contraindicated. Use moxibustion with caution.

GV-16 (fēng fǔ)
WIND'S PALACE

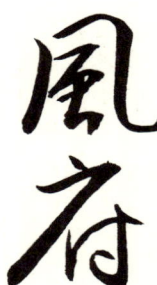

Sea of Marrow point, Intersecting point of the Yang-linking vessel on the Governing vessel.

Located 1 unit above the posterior hairline in the depression inferior to the external occipital protuberance on the posterior midline.

Image:
The name suggests that external pathogenic Wind tends to settle at this point before penetrating deeper.

Functions:
Benefits and clears the Brain, opens the sensory orifices, and dispels Wind, Wind-Cold and Wind-Heat.

> Indications: seizures, mania, hemiplegia, aphasia due to stroke, delirium, suicidal behavior, fear and fright, anxiety, common cold due to Wind-Cold, sensation of heaviness of the head, headache, dizziness, deaf-mutism, blurred vision, sinusitis, epistaxis, and neck stiffness.

Deep needling is contraindicated. Use moxibustion with caution.

GV-17 (nǎo hù)
BRAIN'S DOOR

Intersecting point of Bladder channel on the Governing vessel.

Located on the superior border of the external occipital protuberance on the posterior midline.

Image:
The name refers to this point's function in regulating the Brain and the surrounding tissue and fluid.

Functions:
Benefits and clears the Brain, revives consciousness, dispels Wind, and clears Heat.

> Indications: collapsing syndrome, seizures, mania, vertigo, lassitude and heaviness of the lower extremities due to deficiency, sensation of heaviness of the head, flushed face, occipital headache, blurred vision, and tinnitus.

Use moxibustion with caution.

GV-20 (bǎi huì)
HUNDRED MEETINGS

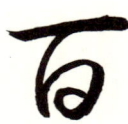
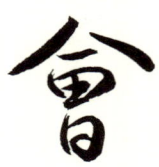

Sea of Marrow point, Intersecting point of the Bladder channel on the Governing vessel.

Located on the midline of the head, halfway between the frontal hairline and the vertex of the external occipital protuberance.

Image:
The name refers to this point's location on the vertex of the head, the Yang pole of the body, and its influence on the various channels which meet here. In Indian philosophy this point is known as the "Thousand Petal Lotus" (*sahasrara-chakra*), the seventh or crown chakra (wheel or circle of energy), suggesting a similar understanding of the energies located at the top of the head.

Functions:
Benefits and clears the Brain, calms the Spirit, and revives consciousness.

> Indications: seizures, insanity, hysteria with insomnia, meningitis, shock, aphasia due to stroke, insomnia, hyperactivity, disturbances of perception and movement, sensation of heaviness of the head, uncontrolled weeping, and forgetfulness.

Spreads Liver Qi, subdues Liver Yang, extinguishes Liver Wind, and dispels Wind.

> Indications: closed-type Wind-stroke, hemiplegia, hypertension, dizziness, parietal headache, vertex headache, deafness, tinnitus, lockjaw, and neck stiffness.

Warms the Yang△ and restores collapsed Yang.△

> Indications: collapsing syndrome due to deficiency, abandoned-type coma, fainting, uterovaginal or rectal prolapse, abnormal uterine bleeding, hemorrhoids, and chronic diarrhea.

Stabilizes the lower orifices,△ regulates and tonifies Qi,△ and calms the Fetus.△

> Indications: restless fetus disorder due to Qi deficiency, infertility, impotence, premature ejaculation, urinary incontinence, hair loss or premature greying, and tinnitus.

GV-23 (shàng xīng)
UPPER STAR

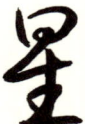

Located 1 unit within the anterior hairline on the midline of the head.

Image:
The name is an indirect reference to the nasal cavity, the orifice associated with the Lungs, which receives cosmic Qi (*da qi*), the Qi from air. (The cosmos is the abode of the stars.) *Upper* refers to this point's position on the top of the head.

Functions:
Clears the nose.

> Indications: nasal blockage, sinusitis, rhinitis, nasal polyps or carbuncles, epistaxis, frontal headache, and voice loss.

Brightens the eyes and clears Heat.

> Indications: redness of the inner canthus, myopia, sudden blindness, eye pain, redness and swelling, tearing due to Wind, facial edema and redness, fever without sweating, and tidal fever.

Moxibustion is contraindicated.

GV-26 (rén zhōng)
MIDDLE OF MAN

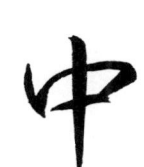

Intersecting point of the Stomach and Large Intestine channels on the Governing vessel.

Located on the philtrum about one-third the distance from the base of the nose to the top of the lip.

Image:
The name refers to the area where the Yin and Yang on the body's midline (Conception and Governing vessels) meet, and to the point from which they can be regulated. *Ren zhong* is also a term for the philtrum.

Functions:
Revives consciousness, calms the Spirit, clears the Brain and Heat, dispels Wind and Wind-Phlegm, and restores collapsed Yang.

    Indications: closed-type Wind-stroke, collapsing syndrome, seizures, shock, heatstroke, hysteria with fainting, facial swelling due to Wind, excessive thirst, eye muscle twitches and cramps, lockjaw, toothache, deviated mouth due to Wind-stroke, and depression with uncontrolled weeping.

Regulates the Governing vessel, strengthens the back, relaxes the sinews, and alleviates pain.

    Indications: convulsions, muscular tetany, all acute spinal pain or muscle spasms, and acute lower back pain or stiffness.

Clears the nose.

    Indications: all nasal disorders including nasal blockage, rhinitis, and epistaxis.

Transforms Heart Phlegm.
> Indications: chest pain and palpitations, distention and heaviness of the chest due to Phlegm.

Moxibustion is contraindicated.

EX-1 (M-HN-3) *(yìn táng)*
SEAL HALL

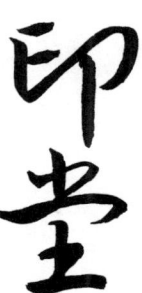

Located on the midline between the medial ends of the two eyebrows.

Image:
Hall refers to this point's area of influence, the inner cranium which stores the mind; *seal* refers to the location, named after an ancient tradition of placing a red mark between the eyebrows (as seen on temple deities) to represent wisdom and enlightenment. This practice, which originated in India, was transmitted to China with Buddhism. *Yin tang* is now a term for the area between the eyebrows.

Functions:
Calms the Spirit, dispels Wind, and clears Heat.
> Indications: insanity, febrile convulsions, convulsions during pregnancy, childhood convulsions, hypertension, frontal headache, vomiting, dizziness, fainting due to blood loss, insomnia, and eye soreness and redness.

Clears the nose.
> Indications: all nasal disorders including nasal blockage, rhinitis, and epistaxis.

EX-2 (M-HN-9) (tài yáng)
SUN

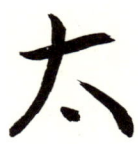

Located in the depression 1 unit posterior to the midpoint between the lateral tip of the eyebrow and the outer canthus.

Image:
The name refers to this point's location in an area on the face which was thought to reveal one's vitality. Traditional diagnosis involved observation of the color of the skin around this point. *Tai yang* is also a term for the temples.

Functions:
Brightens the eyes, dispels Wind and Wind-Heat, clears Heat, and extinguishes Liver Wind.

> Indications: febrile convulsions, common cold with headache, hypertension due to Yang excess, unilateral headache, facial paralysis, trigeminal neuralgia, dizziness due to Liver Wind excess, upper body erysipelas due to Wind-Heat, conjunctivitis, optic nerve atrophy, and sudden blindness.

EX-3 (M-HN-14) *(bí tōng)*
NOSE PASSAGE

Located in the depression below the nasal bone at the superior end of the nasolabial sulcus.

Image:
The name refers to this point's function of opening and regulating the nasal passages.

Functions:
Clears the nose.
> Indications: all nasal and sinus problems including allergic rhinitis, sinusitis, and nasal polyps.

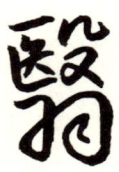
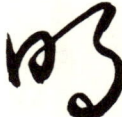

EX-4 (M-HN-13) *(yì míng)*
SHIELDING BRIGHTNESS

Located 1 unit posterior to TB-17 behind the ear.

Image:
The name refers to this point's therapeutic function of removing obstruction to vision, light, or brightness.

Functions:
Calms the Spirit and brightens the eyes.
> Indications: mumps, cataract, myopia, night blindness, atrophy of the optic nerve, insomnia, vertigo, and headache.

Benefits the ears.
> Indications: tinnitus and diminished hearing.

EX-5 (N-BW-21) (ān mián)
PEACEFUL SLEEP

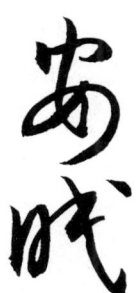

Located midway between G-20 and TB-17.

Image:
The name refers to this point's function of calming the mind and improving the quality of sleep.

Functions:
Calms the Spirit and clears the Brain.

Indications: hysteria, mania, hypertension with insomnia and restlessness, hyperthyroidism with dream-disturbed sleep, deafness, convulsions, insomnia, palpitations, headache, dizziness, and withdrawal symptoms due to drug addiction.

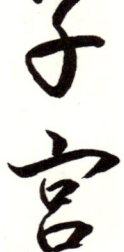

EX-6 (M-CA-18) *(zǐ gōng)*
WOMB

Located 3 units lateral to CV-3.

Image:
The name refers to this point's area of influence.

Functions:
Regulates menstruation, clears Heat, and transforms Damp-Heat.
> Indications: pelvic inflammatory disease, cystitis, infertility, irregular menstruation, menorrhagia, and dysmenorrhea.

Raises the middle Qi.
> Indications: uterine prolapse.

EX-7 (M-BW-1) *(dìng chuǎn)*
STOP WHEEZING

Located 0.5 unit lateral to GV-14.

Image:
The name refers to this point's function.

Functions:
Diffuses Lung Qi.

Indications: bronchitis, asthma, pertussis, cough, neck stiffness, and urticaria.

Local effect: upper back and shoulder pain.

EX-8 (M-BW-24) (yāo yǎn)
LUMBAR'S APERTURE

Located in the depression approximately 3 to 4 units lateral to the spinous process of the third lumbar vertebra.

Image:
The name refers to this point's location in the depression or aperture of the lumbar region.

Functions:
Strengthens the lower back.
> Indications: lower back pain, stiffness or arthritis and acute lower back trauma.

Regulates menstruation.
> Indications: irregular menstruation, ovarian pain, and dysmenorrhea.

EX-9 (M-BW-25)
(shí qī zhuī xià)
BELOW 17 VERTEBRAE

Located inferior to the spinous process of the fifth lumbar vertebra.

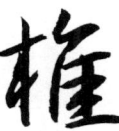

Image:
The name refers to this point's location below the fifth lumbar vertebra; *seventeen* refers to the twelve thoracic and five lumbar vertebrae.

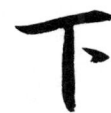

Functions:
Benefits the lower back and regulates the lower Burner.

Indications: traumatic paraplegia, infantile paralysis, anal disorders including hemorrhoids, lumbosacral pain and stiffness, sciatica, functional uterine bleeding, dysmenorrhea, and dysuria.

EX-10 (M-BW-35)
(huá tuó jiā jǐ)
HUA TUO BILATERAL SPINAL POINTS

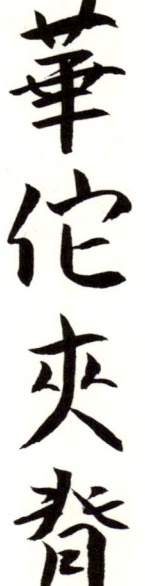

A group of points located about 0.5 to 1 unit lateral to the inferior end of the spinous processes of the cervical, thoracic and lumbar vertebrae.

Image:
These points are named after the famous Han dynasty physician Hua Tuo, who is credited with first using them. In theory, these points are connected by way of the Connecting channels from the Governing vessel to the Bladder channel. Their main function is to facilitate free and smooth Qi circulation through these channels. Stimulating the points lets Qi excess out through the Bladder channel. Their therapeutic functions are basically the same as those of the Governing vessel points.

Functions:
Benefits the back and joints, restores Qi and Blood flow, and strengthens and relaxes the sinews.

> Indications: all internal organ disorders and symptoms, problems of the spine, the adjacent tissues and the extremities (including atrophy syndrome).

Spinal point areas of influence: C1-C4 head region; C1-C7 neck region; C4-C7 upper extremities; C7-T9 chest cavity; T8-L5 abdominal cavity; T11-L5 lumbosacral region; L2-S2 lower extremities; L2-S4 pelvic cavity.

EX-11 (M-UE-9) *(sì fèng)*
FOUR SEAMS

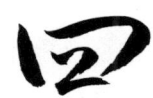
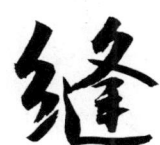

Located on the palmar surface in the transverse creases of the proximal interphalangeal joints of the four fingers (excluding the thumb).

Image:
The name refers to the points' location in the proximal transverse crease of the fingers. *Four* refers to the number of points on each hand.

Functions:
Reduces digestive stagnation, facilitates Qi and Blood flow.
    Indications: childhood nutritional impairment and pertussis.

Expels parasites.
    Indications: intestinal parasites.

Local effect: finger pain due to arthritis.

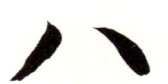

EX-12 (M-UE-22) (bā xié)
EIGHT EVILS

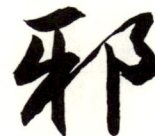

Located on the dorsum of the hand on the web between each finger.

Image:
The name suggests the points' function of clearing away external pathogenic influences or *evils*. The number *eight* refers to the number of points on both hands.

Functions:
Alleviates exterior conditions, dispels Wind, clears Heat, and relaxes the sinews.

> Indications: various localized disorders of the fingers including arthritis, numbness and muscular spasm, upper extremity gangrene, snake bite, headache, toothache, eye pain, neck stiffness, and sore throat.

EX-13 (M-UE-1) *(shí xuān)*
TEN DRAININGS

Located on the middle of the tip of each finger about 0.1 unit from the fingernail.

Image:
The name refers to the points' ability to drain excess Heat from the body. The number *ten* refers to the number of points on both hands.

Functions:
Revives consciousness, clears Heat° and Summerheat.°

> Indications: insanity, febrile diseases, febrile convulsions, childhood convulsions, closed-type coma, stroke, heatstroke, seizures, shock, and sore throat.

Local effect: numbness of the fingertips, paralysis and weakness of the hands.

EX-14 (M-UE-48)
(jiān nèi líng)
SHOULDER'S INNER TOMB

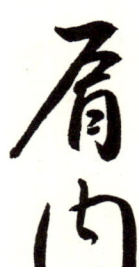

With the arm slightly abducted, located midway between the end of the anterior axillary fold and LI-15.

Image:
The name refers to this point's location on the anterior medial aspect of the shoulder and its ability to restore joint mobility. *Tomb* refers to the shoulder joint and its surrounding deep tissue.

Functions:
Benefits the shoulders, relaxes the sinews, and dispels Wind.

> Indications: pain, atrophy, inflammation and inhibited movement of the shoulder, frozen shoulder, and paralysis of the upper extremities.

EX-15 (M-LE-8) *(bā fēng)*
EIGHT WINDS

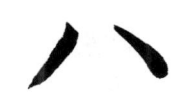
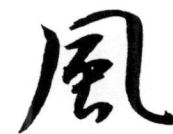

Located on the dorsum of the foot, on the web between each toe, proximal to the margin of the web.

Image:
The name refers to the points' function of dispelling Wind and other external pathogenic influences that are carried by Wind. *Eight* refers to the number of points on both feet.

Functions:
Releases exterior conditions, dispels Wind, clears Heat, and transforms Damp-Heat.

>Indications: malarial disorders, peripheral neuritis, snake bite, headache, toothache, stomachache, lower-leg swelling and lack of circulation, and gangrene of the lower leg and foot.

Local effect: foot and toe disorders including arthritis, numbness, paralysis, muscular spasm and joint problems.

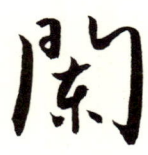
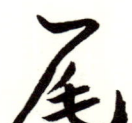

EX-16 (M-LE-13) *(lán wěi)*
APPENDIX

Located 2 units distal to S-36.

Image:
The name refers to this point's area of influence.

Functions:
Regulates the Intestines and transforms Damp-Heat (especially Intestinal).

> Indications: acute and chronic appendicitis, severe lower abdominal pain and cramps, epigastric pain, and indigestion.

Local effect: lower extremity arthritis, pain, and paralysis.

EX-17 (M-LE-23) *(dǎn náng)*
GALLBLADDER

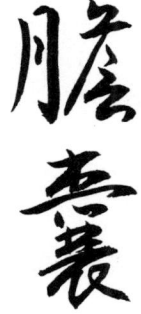

Located 1 unit distal to G-34.

Image:
The name refers to this point's area of influence.

Functions:
Regulates the Gallbladder and transforms Damp-Heat (especially Gallbladder).
    Indications: acute and chronic cholecystitis, biliary colic, and hypochondriac pain.

Expels (Gallbladder) stones and parasites.
    Indications: stones and roundworm in the bile duct.

Local effect: lower extremity pain, paralysis and weakness.

CHAPTER 4

Repertory of Traditional Functions

DIFFERENTIATION	FUNCTION	PRIMARY POINTS	SECONDARY POINTS
Ancestral Qi	Tonifies	L-1, CV-17	B-13, B-15, K-27
Back	Benefits	B-10, B-60, GV-26, EX-10 (M-HN-20)	B-2, B-29, K-7, GV-7, GV-9~10
Bladder	Regulates	S-28, B-28, B-39, CV-3	K-5, K-7, CV-2
Blood	Contains△	Sp-1, B-17, Liv-1	S-30, B-20, Liv-5, CV-2
	Regulates	S-30, Sp-10, B-17, Liv-13	S-25, S-36,△ Sp-8, Sp-21, H-2, B-24, B-43,△ B-60, B-67, CV-12
	Tonifies	Sp-6,△ Sp-10,△ B-17, Liv-8	S-36,△ Sp-8, B-20, B-43, K-3,△ CV-4,△ CV-6△
Blood Dryness	Nourishes	Sp-6	Sp-10, B-17, B-20, Liv-8
Blood flow	Facilitates	Sp-6, H-6, B-17	Sp-1, Sp-10, B-11
Blood, Heat in the	Cools	LI-11, Sp-6, Sp-10, H-7, B-40,○ Liv-3, CV-6	L-6, L-10, H-6, H-9, B-15~18, K-2, K-8, K-10, P-3,○ P-4~5, P-7~8, Liv-2, CV-3, CV-7, GV-1
Blood or Blood stasis	Invigorates	LI-11, Sp-6, Sp-8, Sp-10, B-60, Liv-13	S-30, Sp-4, H-6, B-17, B-31~34, P-2, P-6, Liv-2~3, Liv-8
Bones	Benefits	B-11, G-39, GV-4△	
Brain	Benefits	H-7, B-23,△ K-3, GV-16, GV-17, GV-20	H-3, H-5, B-15, B-44, GV-4

Using the Repertory | The superscript symbol △ indicates moxibustion.
The superscript symbol ○ indicates bloodletting.
The symbol ~ indicates 2 or more consecutive points.

DIFFERENTIATION	FUNCTION	PRIMARY POINTS	SECONDARY POINTS
Brain, CONT.	Clears	H-6~7, P-6~7, GV-26	S-41, Sp-1, Sp-4, H-9, SI-3, SI-5, SI-7, B-15, K-4, P-8, TB-10, CV-1, GV-4, GV-14~17, GV-20, EX-5 (M-HN-18)
Chest	Expands	L-1, L-5, B-13, P-6, CV-17	L-8, S-18, Sp-21, H-1~2, SI-11, B-11~12, B-14~16, B-43~44, K-27, P-1~3, P-5, P-7, TB-6, Liv-14, CV-15, GV-10, GV-11~12
Cold (exterior)	Dispels△	L-7, S-6, B-12, B-13, B-60, G-20~21, G-30~31, G-34	LI-4, S-2~4, S-7, S-31~32, S-35~36, S-38, SI-12, SI-18, B-2, B-10~11, B-29, B-62, TB-14, TB-17, TB-21, G-2, G-12, G-14, G-29, G-33, CV-24, GV-2
Cold (interior)	Warms△	S-36, Sp-6, B-23, K-3, CV-4, CV-6, CV-8, CV-12, GV-4	S-25, B-20, B-25~26, K-2, K-27, Liv-13, CV-2, CV-5, CV-9, CV-13, GV-3. Lower Burner: S-29
Collapsed Yang	Restores	LI-4, S-36, CV-8, GV-4, GV-20	L-11, B-43, K-1, P-9, CV-4,△ CV-6,△ GV-26
Collapsed Yin	Restores	K-3, K-7, CV-6	CV-4, GV-14
Conception vessel	Regulates	L-7	CV-1, CV-6
Consciousness	Revives	L-11, LI-1, K-1, GV-26	H-9, SI-1, B-40, P-8~9, TB-1, CV-1, GV-17, GV-20, EX-13 (M-UE-1)

DIFFERENTIATION	FUNCTION	PRIMARY POINTS	SECONDARY POINTS
Dampness	Dries △	S-36, S-40, B-20~21, CV-8	S-25, Sp-6, CV-4~7, GV-4
	Resolves	Sp-6, Sp-9, CV-4, CV-9	B-22~23, B-26~27, B-52, G-25, CV-6~7
	Transforms	S-25, S-40, Liv-13, CV-12	LI-7, S-31~32, S-36, S-43, Sp-3~4, B-20~21, B-49, P-6, G-29~31, G-33, CV-10~11, CV-13, CV-24
Damp-Cold	Dries △	S-25, S-36, Sp-6, CV-4, CV-8, CV-12. Intestines: B-25	S-40, B-20~21, B-26, CV-5, CV-6~7, GV-3~4
Damp-Heat	Resolves	B-39. Bladder: B-28. Intestines: B-25. Lower Burner: CV-3~4. Spleen-Stomach: Sp-9	B-26, CV-6~7. Liver-Gallbladder: G-36. Lower Burner: B-27, B-54. Spleen-Stomach: Sp-6
	Transforms	S-40, CV-12. Bladder & Intestines: B-40. Intestines: S-25, S-37. Liver-Gallbladder: B-19, G-34, Liv-8, Liv-13. Lower Burner: G-26. Spleen-Stomach: CV-12	LI-3~5, LI-11, S-36, S-39, S-44~45, Sp-3, Sp-5, Sp-12, SI-4, B-20~21, B-49, B-59, B-67, K-6~7, P-8, G-24, G-28, G-37~39, G-41, Liv-6, CV-10~11, CV-13, EX-6 (M-CA-18), EX-15 (M-LE-8). Gallbladder: EX-17 (M-LE-23). Intestines: Sp-15, EX-16 (M-LE-13). Liver-Gallbladder: B-18, G-40, Liv-3~4, Liv-14, GV-9. Lower Burner: S-28~29, H-8, B-30~35, K-8, G-27, Liv-1~2, Liv-5. Spleen-Stomach: Sp-4
Damp-Summer-heat	Resolves	Sp-9	
	Transforms	S-40, B-40	LI-11, P-6, G-34

DIFFERENTIATION	FUNCTION	PRIMARY POINTS	SECONDARY POINTS
Diaphragm	Benefits	B-17, P-6	B-16, P-4, CV-14~15
Digestive stagnation	Reduces	S-25, S-36, Sp-4, Sp-15, Liv-13, CV-12	LI-10, S-21, Sp-2~3, Sp-6, B-20~21, CV-8,△ CV-10, EX-11 (M-UE-9)
Dryness	Moistens	L-5 (Lungs), LI-4, Sp-6, K-6, K-7	L-9, LI-6, LI-11, SI-1, B-43, K-3, TB-2, TB-3, TB-4, TB-6
Ears	Benefits	SI-19, B-23, TB-3, TB-17, TB-21, G-2	G-39, EX-4 (M-HN-13)
	Opens	SI-19, TB-21, G-2	S-7, SI-2
Essence	Stabilizes	S-30, B-30,△ CV-2	B-27, B-31~34,△ K-2, Liv-5,△ CV-1
	Tonifies	B-23,△ K-3,△ GV-4△	Sp-6, B-52△
Exterior conditions	Releases	LI-4, LI-11, S-36, B-13, TB-5, G-20, G-34	L-5, SI-3, B-12, EX-12 (M-UE-22), EX-15 (M-LE-8)
Eyes	Brightens	LI-4, S-2, B-1~2, B-18, B-19, G-20, G-37, EX-2 (M-HN-9)	LI-14, S-1, S-8, SI-6, B-23, B-67, TB-23, G-1, G-14, G-41, GV-23, EX-4 (M-LE-8)
	Opens	LI-4, B-2, G-20	B-1, G-37
Fever	Reduces	LI-4, LI-11, GV-14	S-44, B-10
Fire	Clears	LI-4, LI-11, K-1 (Head), GV-14	SI-3, B-1, B-62, K-2, P-6, TB-1, TB-4, TB-6, TB-23, G-1, CV-23, GV-13
Deficiency Fire	Clears	Sp-6, K-3	K-6

DIFFERENTIATION		FUNCTION	PRIMARY POINTS	SECONDARY POINTS
Fluids		Generates	LI-4, S-36, TB-2	S-25, B-17, TB-6, CV-23
Gallbladder		Regulates	G-34, G-40, G-41, Liv-3	B-18~19, G-24, G-35, G-37~39, G-43~44, Liv-14, GV-9, EX-17 (M-LE-23)
Girdle vessel		Regulates	G-26, G-41	
Governing vessel		Regulates	SI-3, GV-1	GV-26
Hard masses		Softens	LI-4, LI-11, S-36, Sp-6, G-21, Liv-13	LI-10, LI-15~16, LI-18, S-9, SI-10, SI-17, B-18~20, TB-10, TB-17, G-40~41, CV-22
Heart		Regulates	H-5, H-7~8, B-15, P-3, P-6~7, CV-14	H-1, H-3~4, H-6, H-9, B-14, B-43~44, P-2, P-4~5, P-8~9, CV-13, CV-15, GV-11
		Tonifies	H-5~7, B-15, P-5~6	B-14, B-43
	Blood	Tonifies	H-6, P-6	H-7, B-15
	Qi	Regulates-Tonifies	H-5, H-7~8, B-15, P-5~6, CV-14	H-3, B-14, B-43~44, P-3~4, P-7~9, CV-13, GV-11
	Yang	Regulates-Tonifies	H-5, H-7, B-15, P-5, P-8	B-14, P-6, P-9, GV-11
	Yin	Tonifies	H-6, P-6	H-7
Heart Fire		Clears	H-8~9, B-15, P-8~9	H-5, H-7, P-5~7
Heart Pathogenic influences		Drains	H-8, SI-3	CV-4
Heart Phlegm		Transforms	S-40, H-7~8, P-5~6	H-6, SI-3, B-15, K-1, CV-14~15, GV-26

DIFFERENTIATION	FUNCTION	PRIMARY POINTS	SECONDARY POINTS
Heat	Clears	L-10~11, LI-1, LI-4, LI-11, S-44, H-7, SI-3, B-10, B-13, B-15, B-18, B-28, P-9, TB-1,° TB-5, G-20, G-34, Liv-3, CV-12, GV-14 Abdominal: S-25. Head: K-1. Upper Burner: L-1	L-5~6, L-9, LI-2~3, LI-5~7, LI-15, LI-20, S-1~2, S-6~8, S-31~32, S-34~36, S-40~43, S-45, Sp-3~4, Sp-10, H-2, SI-1, SI-4~5, SI-7, SI-12, SI-15, SI-17~19, B-1~2, B-11, B-16~17, B-19, B-35, B-40, B-44, B-47, B-57, B-59, B-62~67, K-2, K-8, P-1, P-3~8, TB-2~4, TB-6~8, TB-10, TB-21, TB-23, G-1~2, G-12, G-14, G-21, G-29~31, G-33, G-36~40, G-43~44, Liv-4, CV-1, CV-15, CV-23~24, GV-1, GV-9~10, GV-12~13, GV-17, GV-23, GV-26, EX-6 (M-CA-18), EX-12 (M-EU-22), EX-13° (M-UE-1), EX-15 (M-LE-8). Small Intestine: H-8. Lower Burner: K-10, CV-3. Middle Burner: S-21
	Deficiency Heat	Clears	Sp-6, H-6, K-3, CV-6	H-5, H-7, K-4, K-6, CV-7
Hip	Benefits	G-29~30, G-34	S-31, B-40
Intestines	Moistens	S-25, S-36, Sp-15, B-25	B-26~27, G-27, EX-16 (M-LE-13)
	Regulates	S-25, S-36~37, B-25	LI-10, S-39~40, S-44, Sp-15, B-26~27, P-3, G-27, CV-8,△ GV-1
Joints	Benefits	B-11, G-34	SI-3, SI-6, G-40, EX-10 (M-BW-35)

DIFFERENTIATION		FUNCTION	PRIMARY POINTS	SECONDARY POINTS
Kidneys		Tonifies	Sp-6, B-23, B-52, K-3, K-6, G-25, CV-6, CV-8,△ GV-4	S-36, B-22, B-43,△ K-1~2, K-4~5, K-7~10, K-27, CV-3~5, CV-7, GV-3
	Qi	Stabilizes	Sp-6, B-23,△ B-52,△ CV-4,△ GV-4△	Sp-8, K-2~3, CV-3,△ GV-3
		Tonifies	B-23, K-3, K-7, CV-6	B-52, CV-3, GV-3~4
	Yang	Tonifies	B-23, K-2~3, CV-6, GV-4	S-36, B-22, B-43, B-52, K-7, K-27, G-25, CV-3~5, CV-7, GV-3
	Yin	Tonifies	Sp-6, K-1, K-3, K-6	B-43, B-52, K-7, K-10, G-25, CV-4
Knee		Benefits	S-35~36, B-23, B-40, G-34, GV-3	B-26, K-10, G-33, Liv-8
Labor		Expedites	LI-4, Sp-6, B-60	B-31~34, B-67, K-6, G-21
Lactation		Expedites	S-18, S-36, B-20, P-6, CV-17	S-1, B-16, P-1, TB-6, Liv-14
		Facilitates	SI-1, P-6, Liv-3, CV-17	S-18, SI-11, P-1, G-21, G-41, Liv-14
Large Intestine		Moistens	LI-4, LI-11, TB-6	
		Regulates	LI-4, LI-11, TB-6	LI-3, LI-7, Sp-3, B-57
Liver		Regulates	B-18, G-34, G-40~41, Liv-2~3, Liv-14	Sp-6, B-19, B-47, P-6, G-24, G-37, Liv-1, Liv-4~5, Liv-8, Liv-13, GV-9
		Tonifies	B-18, Liv-3, Liv-8	G-34, G-37, Liv-1, Liv-5
	Blood	Regulates-Tonifies	G-34, Liv-1, Liv-3, Liv-8	B-18, G-37, G-40, Liv-5, Liv-13

DIFFERENTIATION		FUNCTION	PRIMARY POINTS	SECONDARY POINTS
Liver	Qi	Regulates	B-18~19, G-34, G-41, Liv-3, Liv-8, Liv-14	B-47, P-6, G-24, G-40, Liv-1~2, Liv-4, Liv-13
		Spreads	B-18, G-34, G-41, Liv-3, Liv-8, Liv-14	B-14, B-47, P-6, G-21, G-24, G-40, Liv-1, Liv-4~6, Liv-13, GV-9, GV-20
	Yang	Regulates	G-34, Liv-2~3	B-18~19, B-47
		Subdues	Sp-6, G-20, Liv-2~3, GV-20	B-18, G-34, G-43~44
	Yin	Regulates-Tonifies	Sp-6, Liv-5	G-37, Liv-3, Liv-13
Liver Fire		Clears	G-20, G-40, Liv-2~3	B-18~19, GV-9
Liver Pathogenic influences		Drains	G-34, Liv-3	Liv-8
Liver Wind		Extinguishes	G-20~21, G-34, G-43, Liv-2~3	G-39, G-41, GV-20, EX-2 (M-HN-9)
Lower back		Strengthens	B-23, B-25, B-28, B-40, GV-3, EX-8 (M-BW-24), EX-9 (M-BW-25)	B-24, B-26~27, B-31~34, B-36~37, B-54, B-57, B-61, G-29, G-30, GV-1~2, GV-4~5
Lower Burner		Regulates	S-25, Sp-6, B-23, CV-4, CV-6	S-36, Sp-3~4, Sp-9, B-26, B-31~34, CV-3, CV-7, EX-9 (M-BW-25)
Lower orifices		Stabilizes	Sp-6, B-30,△ GV-20△	S-30, CV-1, GV-1
Lungs		Regulates	L-1, L-5~7, L-9, LI-11, B-13, CV-17	L-8, L-10~11, LI-4, S-36, B-11~12, B-42~43, K-27, CV-22, GV-12
		Tonifies	L-1, L-9, B-13	L-5, S-36

DIFFERENTIATION	FUNCTION	PRIMARY POINTS	SECONDARY POINTS
Lung Qi, CONT.	Regulates-Tonifies	L-1, L-7, B-13, CV-17	L-9, LI-4, LI-11, S-36, B-12, B-43, CV-22, GV-12
	Diffuses	L-1, L-7, B-13, CV-17	LI-1, LI-18, S-9, S-18, SI-15, B-11~12, B-42, P-1, CV-22, GV-12~13, EX-7 (M-BW-1)
Yin	Tonifies	L-5, L-9	L-1
Lung Fire	Clears	L-11○	L-10, LI-1○
Lung Pathogenic influences	Drains	LI-11, S-40	LI-4, S-36
Menstruation	Regulates	S-29~30, Sp-6, Sp-8, Liv-3, Liv-8, CV-3~4	S-25, Sp-4, Sp-10, B-31~34, K-3, K-5~8, G-26~27, CV-1~2, CV-5, CV-7, EX-6 (M-CA-18), EX-8 (M-BW-24)
Middle Burner	Regulates	S-25, S-36, B-20~21, P-6, CV-12	S-21, Sp-3~4, Sp-5~6, Liv-13
Nose	Clears	LI-4, LI-20, GV-26, EX-1 (M-HN-1), EX-3 (M-HN-14)	S-2, B-2, B-7, B-12, B-67, GV-23
Nutritive Qi	Tonifies	S-36, Sp-10, B-20~21, CV-11~12	S-25, S-30, Sp-15
Pain	Alleviates	LI-4, S-44, TB-5, Liv-3, GV-26	SI-3, B-40, P-6, TB-6, G-34
Parasites	Expels	S-2, S-36	S-25, Sp-15, B-19, EX-11 (M-UE-9)

DIFFERENTIATION	FUNCTION	PRIMARY POINTS	SECONDARY POINTS
Penetrating vessel	Regulates	Sp-4	S-30
Phlegm	Transforms	S-40, B-43, P-6, CV-12, CV-17 (chest)	LI-4, LI-18, SI-15, B-13, TB-6, TB-17, Liv-13, CV-14, CV-22~24
Damp-Phlegm	Transforms	L-7, S-40, B-20	L-9, LI-4, B-13
Dry-Phlegm	Transforms	L-9, LI-4	
Phlegm-Cold	Transforms △	LI-4, B-13, B-43, CV-17	L-7, S-40, B-12, B-20
Phlegm-Heat	Transforms	S-40, CV-17	L-9, SI-15, B-13
Protective Qi	Tonifies	LI-4, S-36	K-7, TB-5, GV-13, GV-14
Pulses	Unblocks	L-9, K-7	
Qi	Regulates	LI-4, S-36, TB-6, G-34, Liv-3, GV-14	S-9, S-25, S-30, S-44, Sp-6, Sp-21, H-2, B-18~19, B-24, B-43, B-59, B-67, P-1, Liv-13, CV-1, CV-12, CV-14, GV-20
	Tonifies	LI-4, S-36, CV-6,△ CV-17	Sp-6,△ B-43, CV-1, CV-4, GV-20 △
Qi flow	Facilitates	LI-4, P-6, TB-6, G-20, GV-14	H-1, B-18, B-36, G-21, G-34, GV-15
Qi and Blood flow	Facilitates	LI-11, S-36, B-60, Liv-3	S-31, Sp-12, Sp-21, EX-10 (M-BW-35), EX-11 (M-UE-9)

DIFFERENTIATION	FUNCTION	PRIMARY POINTS	SECONDARY POINTS
Qi (rebellious)	Redirects downward	S-36, B-13, B-21, P-6, G-24, Liv-3, CV-12, CV-17	L-1, L-5~6, L-9, S-37, S-39, H-9, SI-11, B-14, B-40, B-43, B-47, B-49, B-58, K-4, K-27, P-4, G-21, G-39, CV-11, CV-13~15, CV-22
Middle Qi	Raises	S-30, S-36, Sp-6, CV-12	S-21, S-29, B-20, B-31~34, G-28, CV-2, CV-4, CV-6, EX-6 (M-CA-18)
Sensory orifices	Opens	B-10, TB-1, G-20, G-44	L-9, LI-4, SI-1, SI-5, TB-3, TB-8, TB-17, GV-16
Shoulder	Benefits	LI-15, S-38, TB-14, G-21, EX-14 (M-UE-48)	LI-11, LI-16, SI-9~10, SI-12, SI-15
Sinews	Relaxes	LI-4, SI-3, B-11, B-40, B-60, B-62, TB-5, G-20, G-29~31, G-34, Liv-3, GV-14, GV-26, EX-10 (M-BW-35)	LI-14, LI-15, S-2~4 (face), S-6, S-38, SI-4, SI-6, SI-8, B-10, B-37, B-57, B-59, B-61, TB-14, TB-17 (face), G-2, G-25, G-35~36, CV-24 (face), GV-13, EX-12 (M-UE-35), EX-14 (M-UE-48)
	Strengthens	TB-5, G-34	B-10, G-30, EX-10 (M-BW-35)
Small Intestine	Regulates	CV-9	CV-4
Source Qi	Tonifies	B-23, B-52,△ K-3,△ CV-6, GV-4	S-36, Sp-4, CV-4~5

DIFFERENTIATION		FUNCTION	PRIMARY POINTS	SECONDARY POINTS
Spirit		Calms	Sp-1, H-5, H-7, SI-3, B-15, B-43, K-1, K-6, P-6~7, GV-20, GV-26, EX-1 (M-HN-1), EX-5 (N-HN-22)	L-11, LI-5, S-40~42, S-45, Sp-4, H-3~4, H-6, H-8, SI-5, SI-7, SI-19, B-44, B-62, B-64~66, K-4, K-9, P-4~5, TB-10, G-12, Liv-2, CV-1, CV-13~15, GV-1, GV-4, GV-11~14, EX-4 (M-HN-13)
Spleen		Regulates	S-36, Sp-3~4, Sp-6, Sp-9, B-20~21, Liv-13, CV-12	S-21, S-25, Sp-1~2, Sp-5, Sp-8, Sp-10, Sp-15, B-17, B-49, CV-8,△ CV-9~11, CV-13, GV-5, GV-7
		Strengthens	S-36, Sp-3~4, B-20~21, Liv-13	S-21, Sp-5~6, B-49, CV-8,△ CV-11~12
		Tonifies	S-36, Sp-1, Sp-6, Sp-9, B-20~21, CV-8	Sp-8, B-17, Liv-13, CV-12, GV-5
	Qi	Regulates-Tonifies	S-36, Sp-3~4, Sp-6, Liv-13, CV-12	S-25, Sp-2, Sp-8, Sp-10, Sp-15, B-17, B-20~21, B-49, CV-8,△ GV-5
	Yang	Regulates-Tonifies	S-36, Sp-1, Sp-6, Sp-9, B-20, CV-8△	S-21, S-25, Sp-2~4, B-21, B-49, Liv-13, CV-12, GV-5
Stomach		Regulates	S-21, S-25, S-36, S-41, S-44, Sp-3~4, Sp-6, B-20~21, P-6, CV-12	LI-10, S-34, S-37~40, S-42~43, S-45, Sp-2, Sp-5, Sp-9, B-18~19, B-47, B-49, K-27, P-3, P-5, P-7, G-24, Liv-13, CV-8,△ CV-9~11, CV-13~14, GV-5, GV-7
	Qi	Regulates	S-36, S-44, Sp 4, B-21, CV-12	S-21, S-25, S-34, S-41, Sp-2, Sp-3, Sp-6, B-19, B-20, B-47, B-49, CV-8,△ CV-10, CV-11

DIFFERENTIATION	FUNCTION	PRIMARY POINTS	SECONDARY POINTS
Yin	Regulates	S-36, Sp-9, CV-12	S-25, Sp-3, B-20
Stomach Fire	Clears	S-41, S-44, CV-12	S-40, S-42, B-21, CV-13
Stomach Pathogenic influences	Drains	S-44	S-36
Stones (Gallbladder)	Expels	S-36, P-6, EX-17 (M-LE-23)	G-24
Stones (urinary tract)	Expels	S-28, B-23, CV-3	S-25, S-36, B-22, B-28, G-25, CV-6
Summerheat	Clears	LI-11, B-40,° GV-14	L-11,° LI-4, Sp-10, SI-3, P-7~8, P-9,° EX-13° (M-UE-1)
Sweating	Restrains	LI-4, K-7	
	Stimulates	L-7, LI-4, SI-3, B-13, K-7	L-6, L-10, LI-11, SI-7, B-12, K-3
Throat	Moistens	L-10, LI-4, LI-18, K-6, CV-22, GV-15	L-11, LI-1~3, LI-6~7, S-6, S-9, SI-2, SI-17, TB-1~3, CV-23
Tongue	Benefits	H-7, TB-1, CV-23, GV-15	LI-4, LI-7, H-8, P-9
Triple Burner	Regulates	B-22, B-39, TB-6	TB-5
Upper Burner	Regulates	B-13, CV-17	Liv-1, B-15
Urination	Promotes	Sp-9, B-39, CV-3	Sp-6, B-23, B-31~34

DIFFERENTIATION	FUNCTION	PRIMARY POINTS	SECONDARY POINTS
Water Pathways	Regulates	S-28, Sp-6, B-28, B-39, K-3, K-7, CV-3~4, CV-9	Sp-9, B-22~23, B-27, B-52, G-25, CV-6, CV-8,$^\triangle$ GV-4
Wind	Dispels	LI-4, LI-11, LI-15, S-6, S-31, S-36, SI-3, SI-12, B-10, B-12, B-40, B-60, B-62, TB-5, TB-14, G-20~21, G-29~31, G-34, GV-16, GV-26, EX-2 (M-HN-9), EX-12 (M-UE-22), EX-15 (M-LE-8)	LI-6, LI-14, LI-20, S-1~4, S-7~8, S-32, S-35, S-40~43, SI-7~11, SI-18, B-1~2, B-7, B-11, B-13, B-29, B-57~59, B-61, B-63~67, TB-1~4, TB-6~8, TB-10, TB-17, TB-21, TB-23, G-1~2, G-12, G-14, G-33, G-35, G-37~39, G-44, CV-15, CV-24, GV-2, GV-11~14, GV-17, GV-20, EX-14 (M-UE-44)
Wind-Cold	Dispels	L-7,$^\triangle$ LI-4, B-12~13,$^\triangle$ G-20$^\triangle$	LI-20, B-7,$^\triangle$ B-10~11,$^\triangle$ GV-16
Wind-Dryness	Dispels	L-5, LI-4, TB-6	LI-11, B-13
Wind-Heat	Dispels	LI-4, LI-11, S-44, SI-3, B-13, TB-5, G-20	L-5, L-7, L-10~11, LI-1~2, LI-5, LI-14, LI-20, SI-1~2, SI-4~5, B-7, B-10~12, TB-1, TB-3, TB-6, GV-13, GV-16, EX-2 (M-HN-9)
Wind-Phlegm	Dispels	S-40, H-7, B-15, GV-26	SI-3, B-10, P-6, G-34
Womb	Calms	Sp-6, B-67, K-3, Liv-3	S-36, Sp-10, B-40, P-6, G-25, CV-6, CV-12, GV-4, GV-20$^\triangle$
Yang	Warms$^\triangle$	B-23, CV-8, GV-4, GV-20	B-43, G-25, CV-4, CV-5, CV-6, CV-17

DIFFERENTIATION	FUNCTION	PRIMARY POINTS	SECONDARY POINTS
Yang-heel vessel	Regulates	B-62	
Yang-linking vessel	Regulates	TB-5	
Yin	Enriches	L-9, Sp-6, H-6, K-3, Liv-5, CV-4, CV-6	B-1, B-17, K-1, K-7
Yin-heel vessel	Regulates	K-6	
Yin-linking vessel	Regulates	P-6	K-9

APPENDIX I

Character Dictionary

CHARACTER	MEANING	POINT NAME
Ān 安	1. calm, **peaceful**, quiet, tranquil 2. safe, secure 3. satisfied 4. in good health 5. install 6. fix	EX-5 (N-BW-21) *(an mian)*
Bā 八	eight	B-31-34 *(ba liao)*, EX-12 (M-UE-22) *(ba xie)*, EX-15 (M-LE-8) *(ba feng)*
Bái 白	1. **bright, clear, pure, white** 2. [Taoist] a state of emptiness or clear consciousness	S-2 *(si bai)*, Sp-1 *(yin bai)*, Sp-3 *(tai bai)*, B-30 *(bai huan shu)*, G-14 *(yang bai)*
Bǎi 百	1. numerous 2. **one hundred**	GV-20 *(bai hui)*

Using this Dictionary | Bold type indicates terms (or their derivatives) used in chapter 3.
[ ] indicate derivation or usage.
( ) indicate homonyms or variant pronunciations.
[TCM] refers to Traditional Chinese Medicine.

CHARACTER	MEANING	POINT NAME
Bāo 包	1. protuberance, swelling 2. gestation 3. bundle up, **envelop**, wrap 4. contain, enclose 5. assure	Sp-21 (da bao)
Bí 鼻	nose	S-35 (du bi), EX-3 (M-HN-14) (bi tong)
Bì 臂	upper arm	LI-14 (bi nao)
Bì 髀	1. **hips** 2. buttocks	S-31 (bi guan)
Biān 邊	1. edge, margin, rim, side 2. border, **frontier**, limit	B-54 (zhi bian)
Bīn 賓	1. **guest**, visitor 2. (with the bone radical, 4th tone) kneecap 3. trust in 4. acknowledge 5. submit	K-9 (zhu bin)
Bǐng 秉	1. grasp, **hold** 2. control, maintain	SI-12 (bing feng)
Cān 參	1. attend, **take part in** 2. (pronounced shen) root (ren shen or ginseng) 3. refer 4. consult 5. pay respects to 6. impeach an official before the emperor	B-61 (pu can)
Cāng 倉	1. barn, **granary**, storehouse	S-4 (di cang)
Cháng 長	1. **long time** 2. regular, steady 3. forté, strength 4. grow	GV-1 (chang qiang)
Cháng 腸	Intestines	B-25 (da chang shu), B-27 (xiao chang shu)

CHARACTER	MEANING	POINT NAME
Chē 車	1. cart, **vehicle** 2. machine	S-6 (jia che)
Chéng 承	1. **bear**, carry, **support** 2. **contain**, hold 3. undertake 4. order 5. offer 6. contract 7. **receive** 8. enjoy	S-1 (cheng qi), B-36 (cheng fu), B-57 (cheng shan), CV-24 (cheng jiang)
Chí 池	1. an enclosed space with raised sides 2. moat, pond, **pool**	LI-11 (qu chi), P-1 (tian chi), TB-4 (yang chi), G-20 (feng chi)
Chǐ 尺	1. **unit of measurement** based on the span of a man's hand (10 cun = 1 chi) 2. [TCM] the length of the forearm from the middle pulse position to the internal elbow crease 3. [TCM] the proximal pulse	L-5 (chi ze)
Chōng 衝	1. important or strategic place, **thoroughfare** 2. [TCM] the Penetrating vessel 3. assault, **break through, penetrate, rush** 4. flush, pour boiling water onto, rinse	S-30 (qi chong), S-42 (chong yang), Sp-12 (chong men), H-9 (shao chong), P-9 (zhong chong), TB-1 (guan chong), Liv-3 (tai chong)
Chuǎn 喘	1. breathe heavily, gasp for air, **wheeze** 2. asthma	EX-7 (M-BW-1) (ding chuan)
Dà 大	1. **big, great, large,** major 2. eldest 3. heavy	Sp-2 (da du), Sp-15 (da heng), Sp-21 (da bao), B-11 (da zhu), B-25 (da chang shu), K-4 (da zhong), P-7 (da ling), Liv-1 (da dun), GV-14 (da zhui)

CHARACTER	MEANING	POINT NAME
Dài 带	1. belt, **girdle**, ribbon, tape 2. tire 3. area, belt, zone 4. bring up, look after 5. bring, take 6. lead	G-26 (*dai mai*)
Dǎn 膽	Gallbladder	B-19 (*dan shu*), EX-17 (M-LE-23) (*dan nang*)
Dào 道	1. method, **path**, road, **way** 2. Taoism	S-28 (*shui dao*), H-4 (*ling dao*), G-28 (*wei dao*), GV-11 (*shen dao*), GV-13 (*tao dao*)
Dì 地	**earth**, field, land, soil	S-4 (*di cang*), Sp-8 (*di ji*)
Dìng 定	1. certain, definite, sure 2. established 3. calm, **stable** 4. decide, fix, set	EX-7 (M-BW-1) (*ding chuan*)
Dū 都	1. **capital**, metropolis 2. gathering place	Sp-2 (*da du*), Liv-6 (*zhong du*)
Dū 督	1. watch over 2. inspect 3. **govern**, rule	B-16 (*du shu*)
Dú 犢	calf (animal)	S-35 (*du bi*)
Duì 兌	1. barter, convert, exchange 2. (pronounced *yue*) good words that **dispel grief** and arouse joy	S-45 (*li dui*)
Dūn 敦	1. honest, **sincere**, true 2. thick	Liv-1 (*da dun*)
Ěr 耳	1. **ear** 2. along side 3. merely, only	TB-21 (*er men*)
Èr 二	two	LI-2 (*er jian*)

CHARACTER	MEANING	POINT NAME
Fēi 飛	1. accidental, unexpected 2. groundless, unfounded 3. **fly**, flutter in the air, hover 4. dash, race swiftly	B-58 (*fei yang*)
Fèi 肺	Lungs	B-13 (*fei shu*)
Fēn 分	1. (4th tone) part, component; lot, share; function, duty 2. one-tenth (10 *fen* = 1 *cun*) 3. differentiate, discern, distinguish 4. allot, assign, **divide**, separate	CV-9 (*shui fen*)
Fēng 豐	**abundant**, copious, lush, plentiful	S-40 (*feng long*)
Fēng 風	1. **wind** 2. custom, habit 3. rumor 4. reputation	SI-12 (*bing feng*), B-12 (*feng men*), TB-17 (*yi feng*), G-20 (*feng chi*), G-31 (*feng shi*), GV-16 (*feng fu*), EX-15 (M-LE-8) (*ba feng*)
Fēng 封	1. fief 2. territory 3. seal up, **blockade** 4. appoint to an office 5. confer a title	Liv-4 (*zhong feng*)
Fèng 縫	crack, crevice, fissure, **seam**	EX-11 (M-UE-9) (*si feng*)
Fū 跗	1. **tarsal** 2. instep	B-59 (*fu yang*)
Fú 伏	1. hot season, dog days 2. humbled 3. **prostrate** 4. hide 5. ambush 6. serve 7. admit defeat or guilt	S-32 (*fu tu*)
Fú 扶	1. help, **relieve, support** 2. prop up 3. four fingers' breadth	LI-18 (*fu tu*), B-36 (*cheng fu*)

CHARACTER	MEANING	POINT NAME
Fǔ 府	1. archives, treasury 2. **palace** 3. seat of government 4. storehouse 5. [TCM] (with the flesh radical) a Yang Organ	L-1 (*zhong fu*), H-8 (*shao fu*), K-27 (*shu fu*)
Fǔ 輔	1. minister 2. assist, help	G-38 (*yang fu*)
Fù 復	1. go back, **repeat**, return, turn around 2. recover 3. resume	K-7 (*fu liu*)
Gān 肝	Liver	B-18 (*gan shu*)
Gāo 膏	1. fat, grease, ointment, paste 2. **fatty tissue** 3. disease 4. defect, fault 5. ill, sick	B-43 (*gao huang shu*)
Gé 膈	diaphragm	B-17 (*ge shu*)
Gēn 根	base, **root**, source	S-18 (*ru gen*)
Gōng 公	1. **husband's father** 2. duke, official 3. male (animal) 4. common, public	Sp-4 (*gong sun*)
Gōng 宮	1. **palace** 2. uterus, **womb** 3. castration 4. first note in the ancient musical scale corresponding to the earth phase	SI-19 (*ting gong*), P-8 (*lao gong*), EX-6 (M-CA-18) (*zi gong*)
Gōu 溝	channel, **drain, ditch,** moat, ravine, trench	TB-6 (*zhi gou*), Liv-5 (*li gou*)
Gǔ 谷	ravine, **valley**	LI-4 (*he gu*), S-43 (*xian gu*), SI-2 (*qian gu*), SI-5 (*yang gu*), B-66 (*zu tong gu*), K-2 (*ran gu*), K-10 (*yin gu*)

CHARACTER	MEANING	POINT NAME
Gǔ 骨	1. **bone,** skeleton 2. courage, spirit, spunk	LI-16 (ju gu), SI-4 (wan gu), B-64 (jing gu), B-65 (shu gu), G-12 (wan gu), CV-2 (qu gu)
Guān 關	1. barrier, **border gate,** custom's house, strategic pass 2. crisis, juncture 3. [TCM] the middle pulse 4. **hinge,** joint 5. close, shut	S-7 (xia guan), S-31 (bi guan), B-26 (guan yuan shu), P-6 (nei guan), TB-1 (guan chong), TB-5 (wai guan), G-33 (xi yang guan), CV-4 (guan yuan), GV-3 (yao yang guan)
Guāng 光	1. smooth, glossy 2. bare, naked 3. **brightness, light,** luster 4. glory, honor 5. exhaust, use up 6. alone	G-37 (guang ming)
Guāng 胱	Bladder	B-28 (pang guang shu)
Guī 歸	1. go back, **return** 2. come together, converge	S-29 (gui lai)
Hǎi 海	1. measure word for an accumulation of things or a mass of people 2. **sea**	Sp-10 (xue hai), H-3 (shao hai), SI-8 (xiao hai), B-24 (qi hai shu), K-6 (zhao hai), CV-6 (qi hai)
Hé 合	1. **join,** meet, unite 2. close, shut	LI-4 (he gu)
Héng 橫	crosswise, horizontal, **transverse**	Sp-15 (da heng)
Hòu 後	1. **back,** rear 2. descendants, posterity 3. (homonym) empress, ruler 4. behind 5. afterwards	SI-3 (hou xi)
Hù 户	1. **door,** window 2. family, household	B-42 (po hu), GV-17 (nao hu)

CHARACTER DICTIONARY

CHARACTER	MEANING	POINT NAME
Huán 環	1. bracelet, hoop, **ring** 2. **circumflexus** 3. encircle, surround	B-30 (*bai huan shu*), G-30 (*huan tiao*)
Huāng 肓	region between the heart and diaphragm	B-43 (*gao huang shu*)
Huì 會	1. association, guild, society 2. **assemble, gather,** meet, **reunion** 3. (pronounced *kuai*) collect 4. able to, know how	B-35 (*hui yang*), TB-7 (*hui zong*), G-2 (*ting hui*), CV-1 (*hui yin*), GV-20 (*bai hui*)
Hún 魂	spiritual soul	B-47 (*hun men*)
Jī 機	1. organic 2. machine, **mechanism** 3. crucial point, key link, importance 4. opportunity	Sp-8 (*di ji*)
Jí 極	1. extreme limit, **utmost** point, zenith 2. **pole**	H-1 (*ji quan*), CV-3 (*zhong ji*)
Jĭ 脊	back or **spine**	EX-10 (M-BW-35) (*jia ji*)
Jì 際	1. **border**, edge, limit 2. occasion 3. juncture	L-10 (*yu ji*)
Jiā 夾	bilateral, on both sides	EX-10 (M-BW-35) (*hua tuo jiaji*)
Jiá 頰	jaw	S-6 (*jia che*)
Jiān 間	1. (4th tone) crevice; **interval** 2. intervene, **mediate** 3. **between**	LI-2 (*er jian*), LI-3 (*san jian*), P-5 (*jian shi*), Liv-2 (*xing jian*)

CHARACTER	MEANING	POINT NAME
Jiān 肩	shoulder	LI-15 (*jian yu*), SI-9 (*jian zhen*), SI-15 (*jian zhong shu*), TB-14 (*jian liao*), G-21 (*jian jing*), EX-14 (M-UE-48) (*jian nei ling*)
Jiàn 建	1. (with the man radical) healthy, strong, vigorous 2. establish, found, set up 3. **build**, construct, erect 4. advocate, propose	CV-11 (*jian li*)
Jiāng 漿	sauce, starch, syrup, thick **liquid**	CV-24 (*cheng jiang*)
Jiāo 交	1. **intersection, junction** 2. communication, **intercourse** 3. give to 4. deliver 6. exchange	Sp-6 (*san yin jiao*), K-8 (*jiao xin*), G-35 (*yang jiao*), CV-7 (*yin jiao*)
Jiāo 焦	1. **burned**, charred, parched, scorched 2. melancholy, sad 3. anxious, worried	B-22 (*san jiao shu*)
Jiě 解	1. loosen, separate, undo, untie 2. disperse, **release**	S-41 (*jie xi*)
Jīn 金	1. **gold**, metal 2. [TCM] the metal phase of the five phases	B-63 (*jin men*)
Jīng 京	1. exalted, great, high 2. **capital**, metropolis 3. ten million	B-64 (*jing gu*), G-25 (*jing men*)
Jīng 經	1. [TCM] channel, meridian 2. [weaving] warp 3. canon, classic, scripture 4. menstruation 5. **pass through**, undergo 6. manage, regulate	L-8 (*jing qu*)

CHARACTER DICTIONARY

CHARACTER	MEANING	POINT NAME
Jīng 睛	**eyeball**, iris, pupil	B-1 (jing ming)
Jǐng 井	pit, shaft, **well**	TB-10 (tian jing), G-21 (jian jing)
Jiū 鳩	pigeon, **turtledove**	CV-15 (jiu wei)
Jū 居	1. dwell, **inhabit**, reside 2. remain, stay put	G-29 (ju liao)
Jù 巨	big, **gigantic, great, large**, tremendous, very	LI-16 (ju gu), S-3 (ju liao), S-37 (shang ju xu), S-39 (xia ju xu), CV-14 (ju que)
Jué 厥	1. **absolute**, extreme 2. incurable, terminal	B-14 (jue yin shu)
Kōng 空	1. air, sky 2. hollow, **hole** 3. empty, void 4. in vain, useless	TB-23 (si zhu kong)
Kǒng 孔	**aperture**, hole, opening, orifice	L-6 (kong zui)
Kǒu 口	1. entrance, **gate**, hole, mouth, opening 2. knife blade or edge 3. domestic animals	S-38 (tiao kou)
Kūn 崑	1. **Kunlun mountains** 2. (without the mountain radical) elder brother, posterity	B-60 (kun lun)
Lái 來	1. **come** 2. arrive, reach 3. future	S-29 (gui lai)
Lán 闌	1. end (of the year), late (in the night) 2. exhausted, weary 3. **appendix**, large intestine 4. fence, railing	EX-16 (M-LE-13) (lan wei)

CHARACTER	MEANING	POINT NAME
Láo 勞	1. exhaustion, fatigue 2. **labor**, toil, work 3. bother, trouble 4. (4th tone) reward	P-8 (lao gong)
Lǎo 老	1. aged, **old**, venerable 2. tough (meat) 3. outdated 4. overgrown	SI-6 (yang lao)
Lí 蠡	calabash	Liv-5 (li gou)
Lǐ 里	1. **unit** of linear measure (about one-third of a mile) 2. neighborhood, village 3. a small **route** 4. (homonym) inner, **inside**	LI-10 (shou san li), S-36 (zu san li), H-5 (tong li), CV-11 (jian li)
Lì 歷	1. experience a **passage** of time or events, duration 2. succession, 3. arrange, order	LI-6 (pian li)
Lì 厲	1. harsh, severe, stern 2. cruel, oppressive 3. bad, **evil** 4. a malevolent spirit 5. whetstone 6. sharpen	S-45 (li dui)
Lián 廉	1. honest, incorruptible, **pure** 3. inexpensive	CV-23 (lian quan)
Liáng 梁	1. bridge over a brook (**connecting** two sides) 2. roof beam 3. (with the grain radical) cereal, grain, millet	S-21 (liang men), S-34 (liang qiu)
Liáo 髎	1. **foramen, opening**, hole 2. **joint** 3. **seam**	S-3 (ju liao), SI-18 (quan liao), B-31-34 (ba liao), TB-14 (jian liao), GI (tong zi liao), G-29 (ju liao)
Liè 列	1. **sequence**, series 2. rank and file 3. separate 4. arrange	L-7 (lie que)

CHARACTER DICTIONARY

CHARACTER	MEANING	POINT NAME
Lín 臨	1. near, **on the verge of** 2. face-to-face 3. arrive, reach 4. look at from above, overlook 5. copy, imitate	G-41 (*zu lin qi*)
Líng 靈	1. clever, intelligent 2. effective 3. supernatural 4. soul, **spirit** 5. bier, coffin	H-2 (*qing ling*), H-4 (*ling dao*), GV-10 (*ling tai*)
Líng 陵	1. hill, **mound** 2. **imperial tomb**, mausoleum	Sp-9 (*yin ling quan*), P-7 (*da ling*), G-34 (*yang ling quan*), EX-14 (M-UE-48) (*jian nei ling*)
Liū 溜	1. **current**, stream 2. **flow**	LI-7 (*wen liu*), K-7 (*fu liu*)
Lóng 隆	1. grand, noble 2. **flourishing**, prosperous, thriving 3. sound of thunder	S-40 (*feng long*)
Lǔ 膂	spine	B-29 (*zhong lu shu*)
Lún 崙	Kunlun mountains	B-60 (*kun lun*)
Luò 絡	1. net, web 2. cord, twine 3. [TCM] **connecting channels**	TB-8 (*san yang luo*)
Mài 脈	1. [TCM] **vessel** 2. [TCM] pulse 3. blood vessel	B-62 (*shen mai*), G-26 (*dai mai*)
Mén 門	1. **door**, entrance, **gate** 2. party, school, sect	S-21 (*liang men*), Sp-12 (*chong men*), H-7 (*shen men*), B-12 (*feng men*), B-37 (*yin men*), B-47 (*hun men*), B-63 (*jin men*), P-4 (*xi men*), TB-2 (*ye men*), TB-21 (*er men*), G-25 (*jing men*), Liv-13 (*zhang men*), Liv-14 (*qi men*), CV-5 (*shi men*), GV-4 (*ming men*), GV-15 (*ya men*)

CHARACTER	MEANING	POINT NAME
Mián 眠	1. **sleep** 2. close the eyes 3. hibernate	EX-5 (N-BW-21) (*an mian*)
Míng 明	1. **bright, clear** 2. be clear, obvious 3. open-minded 4. **light** 5. understand	B-1 (*jing ming*), G-37 (*guang ming*), EX-4 (M-HN-13) (*yi ming*)
Mìng 命	1. life, **vitality** 2. destiny, fate 3. command, decree	GV-4 (*ming men*)
Náng 囊	1. **Gallbladder** 2. bag, pocket, sack	EX-17 (M-LE-23) (*dan nang*)
Nǎo 腦	Brain	GV-17 (*nao hu*)
Nào 臑	1. **upper arm** 2. **scapula**	LI-14 (*bi nao*), SI-10 (*nao shu*)
Nèi 内	1. inner, **internal** 2. inside, interior	S-44 (*nei ting*), P-6 (*nei guan*), EX-14 (M-UE-48) (*jian nei ling*)
Páng 膀	Bladder	B-28 (*pang guang shu*)
Pí 脾	Spleen	B-20 (*pi shu*)
Piān 偏	1. be contrary, **deviant** 2. inclined, leaning 3. biased, partial	LI-6 (*pian li*)
Pò 魄	1. **animal soul** 2. [Taoist] life, vigor	B-42 (*po hu*)
Pú 僕	servant	B-61 (*pu can*)
Qī 七	seven	EX-9 (M-BW-25) (*shi qi zhui xia*)

CHARACTER DICTIONARY

CHARACTER	MEANING	POINT NAME
Qī 期	1. expect, **hope** 2. meet, wait 3. date, fixed time period	Liv-14 (qi men)
Qì 氣	1. air, atmosphere, gas, vapor 2. character, spirit 3. odor, smell 4. weather 5. [TCM] **vital energy** 6. anger, enrage	S-30 (qi chong), B-24 (qi hai shu), CV-6 (qi hai)
Qì 泣	1. **tears** 2. cry, sob, weep	S-1 (cheng qi), G-41 (zu lin qi)
Qián 前	1. in front of 2. before, formerly 3. **foreward**, preceding	SI-2 (qian gu)
Qiáng 強	1. **strong**, powerful 2. violent 3. energetic 4. better	GV-1 (chang qiang)
Qiào 竅	**aperture**, cavity, opening, orifice	G-44 (zu qiao yin)
Qīng 青	1. young 2. **green** or blue-green (the natural hue of plants) 3. [TCM] the color corresponding to the wood phase	H-2 (qing ling)
Qīu 丘	**hill, mound**	S-34 (liang qiu), Sp-5 (shang qiu), G-36 (wai qiu), G-40 (qiu xu)
Qū 曲	1. bent, **crooked, curved** 2. false, wrong	LI-11 (qu chi), P-3 (qu ze), Liv-8 (qu quan), CV-2 (qu gu)
Qú 渠	canal, channel, **ditch**, drain	L-8 (jing qu)
Quán 泉	1. fountain 2. **spring**	Sp-9 (yin ling quan), H-1 (ji quan), K-1 (yong quan), K-5 (shui quan), P-2 (tian quan), Liv-8 (qu quan), CV-23 (lian quan)
Quán 顴	cheekbone	SI-18 (quan liao)

CHARACTER	MEANING	POINT NAME
Quē 缺	1. **broken**, defective 2. deficient, imperfect 3. opening, vacancy	L-7 (lie que)
Què 闕	watchtower situated on either side of a palace gate	CV-8 (shen que), CV-14 (ju que)
Rán 然	1. **burn**, light 2. correct, right 3. but, nevertheless	K-2 (ran gu)
Rén 人	1. human being, **man**, people 2. adult, grown up 3. character, personality	S-9 (ren ying), GV-26 (ren zhong)
Rì 日	1. **sun** 2. day, daytime 3. time	G-24 (ri yue)
Róng 容	1. facial expression 2. appearance, looks 3. **receive** 4. contain, hold 5. allow, permit 6. tolerate	SI-17 (tian rong)
Rǔ 乳	1. **breast** 2. milk	S-18 (ru gen)
Sān 三	three	LI-3 (san jian), LI-10 (shou san li), S-36 (zu san li), Sp-6 (san yin jiao), B-22 (san jiao shu), TB-8 (san yang luo)
Shān 山	hill, **mountain**	B-57 (cheng shan)
Shāng 商	1. second note in the ancient Chinese musical scale corresponding to the **metal** phase 2. commerce, trade 3. businessman, merchant, trader 4. consult, discuss	L-11 (shao shang), LI-1 (shang yang), Sp-5 (shang qiu)
Shàng 上	1. **upper** 2. above 3. better, superior 4. board, get on mount	S-37 (shang ju xu), CV-13 (shang wan), GV-23 (shang xing)

CHARACTER DICTIONARY

CHARACTER	MEANING	POINT NAME
Shào 少	1. **young** 2. (3rd tone) few, **less**, little; lack, short	L-11 (shao shang), H-3 (shao hai), H-8 (shao fu), H-9 (shao chong), SI-1 (shao ze)
Shè 舍	1. cottage, **dwelling**, house, hut 2. unit of linear measure equal to 30 li (see li above)	B-49 (yi she)
Shēn 申	1. ninth of the twelve earthly branches 2. explain, express, state. 3. (with the man radical) **extend**, prolong, stretch	B-62 (shen mai)
Shēn 身	1. **body** (human or animal) 2. moral character and conduct 3. body, main part of a structure, trunk 4. oneself, personally	GV-12 (shen zhu)
Shén 神	1. magical, supernatural 2. clever, smart 3. deity, divinity, god 4. mind, **spirit** 5. expression or look	H-7 (shen men), B-44 (shen tang), CV-8 (shen que), GV-11 (shen dao)
Shèn 腎	Kidneys	B-23 (shen shu)
Shí 十	ten	EX-9 (M-BW-25) (shi qi zhui xia), EX-13 (M-UE-1) (shi xuan)
Shí 石	mineral, rock, **stone**	CV-5 (shi men)
Shǐ 使	1. **envoy**, messenger 2. send 3. tell 4. apply, employ, use	P-5 (jian shi)
Shì 市	city, **market**	G-31 (feng shi)
Shì 室	1. **chamber**, room 2. abode, home, household	B-52 (zhi shi)

CHARACTER	MEANING	POINT NAME
Shǒu 手	hand	LI-10 (shou san li)
Shū 樞	1. center, hub, **pivot** 2. **axis**	S-25 (tian shu), G-27 (wu shu), GV-5 (xuan shu), GV-7 (zhong shu)
Shū 俞	1. small boat or primitive barge 2. [TCM] the acupuncture points which convey or contain Qi (**hollow**) 3. (with the cart radical) transport	SI-10 (nao shu), SI-15 (jian zhong shu), B-13 (fei shu), B-14 (jue yin shu), B-15 (xin shu), B-16 (du shu), B-17 (ge shu), B-18 (gan shu), B-19 (dan shu), B-20 (pi shu), B-21 (wei shu), B-22 (san jiao shu), B-23 (shen shu), B-24 (qi hai shu), B-25 (da chang shu), B-26 (guan yuan shu), B-27 (xiao chang shu), B-28 (pang guang shu), B-29 (zhong lu shu), B-30 (bai huan shu), B-43 (gao huang shu), K-27 (shu fu), GV-2 (yao shu)
Shù 束	1. bind, tie 2. control, **restrain**	B-65 (shu gu)
Shuǐ 水	1. **water** 2. liquid 3. river 4. general term for lakes, seas, and rivers	S-28 (shui dao), K-5 (shui quan), CV-9 (shui fen)
Sī 絲	1. threadlike 2. **silk**	TB-23 (si zhu kong)
Sì 四	four	S-2 (si bai), EX-11 (M-UE-9) (si feng)
Sūn 孫	1. **descendants**, posterity 2. grandchild 3. second growth of plants 4. [TCM] the lesser connecting channels	Sp-4 (gong sun)
Tái 臺	1. **platform**, stage, terrace 2. stand, support 3. desk, table	GV-10 (ling tai)

CHARACTER	MEANING	POINT NAME
Tài 太	1. **greatest**, highest, remotest 2. senior, superior 3. excessively, over, too 4. extremely	L-9 (tai yuan), Sp-3 (tai bai), K-3 (tai xi), Liv-3 (tai chong), EX-2 (M-HN-9) (tai yang)
Tán 膻	1. sternum 2. (with the earth radical) **altar**, platform	CV-17 (tan zhong)
Táng 堂	1. court of law 2. **hall** 3. main room of a house 4. the relationship between paternal cousins	B-44 (shen tang), EX-1 (M-HN-3) (yin tang)
Táo 陶	1. contented, happy 2. kiln 3. ceramics, earthenware, pottery 4. make pottery 5. cultivate, **mould**	GV-13 (tao dao)
Tiān 天	1. **heaven**, sky 2. weather 3. nature	S-25 (tian shu), SI-11 (tian zong), SI-17 (tian rong), B-7 (tong tian), B-10 (tian zhu), P-1 (tian chi), P-2 (tian quan), TB-10 (tian jing), CV-22 (tian tu)
Tiáo 條	1. orderly, organized 2. twig 3. measure unit for long and narrow things 4. a long and **narrow** piece or strip 5. article, item 6. northeast wind	S-38 (tiao kou)
Tiào 跳	1. bounce, jump, **leap**, spring 2. beat, move up and down 3. make omissions, skip over	G-30 (huan tiao)
Tīng 聽	1. **hear**, listen 2. heed, obey 3. administer, manage 4. allow	SI-19 (ting gong), G-2 (ting hui)
Tíng 庭	1. court of law 2. front **courtyard** 3. audience hall	S-44 (nei ting)

CHARACTER	MEANING	POINT NAME
Tōng 通	1. coherent, logical 2. fluent, know well, understand thoroughly 3. open, **pass through**, unimpeded 4. clear out, open up 5. go to, lead to, **reach** 6. **communicate, connect**	H-5 (tong li), B-7 (tong tian), B-66 (zu tong gu), EX-3 (M-HN-14) (bi tong)
Tóng 瞳	pupil	G-1 (tong zi liao)
Tóu 頭	1. head 2. **skull**	S-8 (tou wei)
Tū 突	1. abrupt, sudden 2. **chimney** 3. **protrude**, project, stick out 4. charge, dash forward	LI-18 (fu tu), CV-22 (tian tu)
Tù 兔	hare, **rabbit**	S-32 (fu tu)
Wài 外	1. **outer**, outward 2. external, foreign 3. besides, beyond, in addition 4. unofficial	TB-5 (wai guan), G-36 (wai qiu)
Wán 完	1. **complete**, finish 2. intact, whole 3. run out, use up	G-12 (wan gu)
Wǎn 脘	stomach cavity	CV-10 (xia wan), CV-12 (zhong wan), CV-13 (shang wan)
Wàn 腕	wrist	SI-4 (wan gu)
Wéi 維	1. thinking, thought 2. dimension 3. pattern, rule 4. hold together, tie up 5. maintain, **preserve, safeguard**	S-8 (tou wei), G-28 (wei dao)
Wěi 尾	1. **tail** 2. end, rear, stern	CV-15 (jiu wei)

CHARACTER	MEANING	POINT NAME
Wěi 委	1. indirect, roundabout, tactful 2. dispirited, listless 3. appoint, **entrust** 4. cast aside, discard, throw away 5. shift (blame) 6. actually, certainly	B-39 (wei yang), B-40 (wei zhong)
Wèi 胃	Stomach	B-21 (wei shu)
Wēn 温	1. temperature 2. warm, mild, **temperate**	LI-7 (wen liu)
Wǔ 五	five	G-27 (wu shu)
Xī 溪	brook, **stream**	LI-5 (yang xi), S-41 (jie xi), SI-3 (hou xi), K-3 (tai xi), G-43 (xia xi)
Xī 膝	knee	G-33 (xi yang guan)
Xì 郄	1. crack, **crevice**, fissure, gap, space 2. breach (friendship) 3. [TCM] the Accumulating points	H-6 (yin xi), P-4 (xi men)
Xiá 侠	1. **brave,** chivalry 2. hero 3. (without the man radical and pronounced *jia*) place in between, press from both sides	G-43 (xia xi)
Xià 下	1. **below,** under 2. **lower,** inferior 3. alight, descend	S-7 (xia guan), S-39 (xia ju xu), CV-10 (xia wan), EX-9 (M-BW-25) (shi qi zhui xia)
Xiàn 陷	1. pitfall, trap 2. cave in, **sink** 3. frame, incriminate	S-43 (xian gu)
Xiāng 香	1. aromatic, **fragrant**, scented, sweet-smelling 2. [TCM] the odor corresponding to the earth phase 3. perfume, spice	LI-20 (ying xiang)

CHARACTER	MEANING	POINT NAME
Xiǎo 小	1. little, minor, **small** 2. young 3. for a short while	SI-8 *(xiao hai)*, B-27 *(xiao chang shu)*
Xié 邪	1. **evil**, heretical, irregular 2. [TCM] the pathogenic influences (Cold, Dampness, Wind, etc.)	EX-12 (M-UE-22) *(ba xie)*
Xīn 心	1. **Heart** 2. feeling, heart, mind, intention 3. center, core	B-15 *(xin shu)*
Xìn 信	1. true 2. confidence, **faith**, trust 3. letter 4. message, information, 5. arsenic	K-8 *(jiao xin)*
Xīng 星	1. **star** 2. heavenly body	GV-23 *(shang xing)*
Xíng 行	1. makeshift, temporary 2. current, prevalent 3. capable, competent 4. behavior, conduct 5. go on foot, walk 6. **travel** 7. carry out, engage in	Liv-2 *(xing jian)*
Xū 虛	empty, vacant, **void**	S-37 *(shang ju xu)*, S-39 *(xia ju xu)*
Xuān 宣	1. announce, declare, proclaim 2. lead off (liquids), **drain** 3. disseminate, spread	EX-13 (M-UE-1) *(shi xuan)*
Xuán 懸	1. far apart 2. dangerous 3. be solicitous, feel anxious 4. outstanding, unresolved 5. hang, **suspend** 6. imagine	G-39 *(xuan zhong)*, GV-5 *(xuan shu)*
Xuè 血	Blood	Sp-10 *(xue hai)*
Yǎ 瘂	1. dumb, **mute** 2. hoarse	GV-15 *(ya men)*

CHARACTER	MEANING	POINT NAME
Yǎn 眼	1. the eye 2. **aperture**, small hole 3. key point 4. trap 5. [traditional Chinese music] an unaccented beat 6. glance, look	EX-8 (M-BW-24) (*yao yan*)
Yáng 陽	1. [Chinese philosophy] **masculine or positive principle in nature** (opposite of *yin*) 2. [TCM] refers to back, hollow Organs, Qi, upper body 3. sun 4. south face of a mountain, source of a river 5. sunlight, sunshine 6. male genitals	LI-1 (*shang yang*), LI-5 (*yang xi*), S-42 (*chong yang*), SI-5 (*yang gu*), B-35 (*hui yang*), B-39 (*wei yang*), B-58 (*fei yang*), B-59 (*fu yang*), TB-4 (*yang chi*), TB-8 (*san yang luo*), G-34 (*yang ling quan*), G-36 (*yang jiao*), G-38 (*yang fu*), GV-3 (*yao yang quan*), GV-9 (*zhi yang*), EX-2 (M-HN-9) (*tai yang*)
Yǎng 養	1. provide for, **support** 2. grow up, keep, raise 3. give birth to 4. acquire, cultivate 5. convalesce, rest 6. keep in good repair, maintain	SI-6 (*yang lao*)
Yāo 腰	1. **lumbar** 2. small of the back, waist 3. waist (of a garment) 4. middle	GV-2 (*yao shu*), GV-3 (*yao yang guan*), EX-8 (M-BW-24) (*yao yan*)
Yè 液	1. **fluid**, juice, liquid 2. [TCM] body fluids including spittle, sweat, and various secretions	TB-2 (*ye men*)
Yì 意	1. desire, intention 2. [TCM] **intelligence** 3. hint, suggestion, trace 4. idea, meaning 5. opinion, thought 6. anticipate, expect	B-49 (*yi she*)
Yì 翳	1. cover, **screen**, shade 2. [TCM] a slight corneal opacity, nebula 3. cataract	TB-17 (*yi feng*), EX-4 (M-HN-13) (*yi ming*)

CHARACTER	MEANING	POINT NAME
Yīn 陰	1. [Chinese philosophy] **the feminine or negative principle in nature** (opposite of yang) 2. [TCM] refers to front, solid Organs, Blood, lower body 3. moon 4. north face of a mountain, mouth of a river 5. cloudy weather, darkness, shade 6. female reproductive organs	Sp-6 (san yin jiao), Sp-9 (yin ling quan), H-6 (yin xi), B-14 (jue yin shu), B-67 (zhi yin), K-10 (yin gu), G-44 (zu qiao yin), CV-1 (hui yin), CV-7 (yin jiao)
Yīn 殷	1. **abundant**, rich 2. ardent, eager 3. hospitable	B-37 (yin men)
Yǐn 隱	1. concealed, **hidden** 2. dormant, latent	Sp-1 (yin bai)
Yìn 印	1. chop, **seal**, stamp 2. engrave, print 3. conform, tally	EX-1 (M-HN-3) (yin tang)
Yíng 迎	1. **receive, welcome** 2. move toward	LI-20 (ying xiang), S-9 (ren ying)
Yǒng 湧	1. **gush**, pour, surge, well up 2. bubble up, rise	K-1 (yong quan)
Yú 魚	fish	L-10 (yu ji)
Yú 髃	1. **corner**, nook 2. border, outlying place	LI-15 (jian yu)
Yuān 淵	**abyss**, deep pool	L-9 (tai yuan)
Yuán 元	1. first, head, primary 2. chief, principal 3. basic, fundamental 4. (homonym) origin, **source**	B-26 (guan yuan shu), CV-4 (guan yuan)

CHARACTER	MEANING	POINT NAME
Yuè 月	1. round 2. **moon** 3. month	G-24 (ri yue)
Zǎn 攢	1. accumulate, hoard, save 2. (also pronounced cuán) **collect**, gather	B-2 (zan zhu)
Zé 澤	1. damp, moist 2. **marsh**, pool, swamp 3. luster 4. beneficence, favor	L-5 (chi ze), SI-1 (shao ze), P-3 (qu ze)
Zhāng 章	1. chapter, section 2. seal, stamp 3. regulations, rules 4. badge, medal 5. **orderly**, systematically	LI-13 (zhang men)
Zhào 照	1. in the direction of, towards 2. license, permit 3. **illuminate**, shine 4. mirror, reflect 5. take a photograph 6. check against, contrast 7. notify	K-6 (zhao hai)
Zhēn 貞	1. faithful, loyal 2. chastity 3. **integrity** 4. divination	SI-9 (jian zhen)
Zhèng 正	1. honest, straight, upright 2. situated in the middle, **main** 3. principal 4. plus, positive 5. exactly, precisely	SI-7 (zhi zheng)
Zhī 支	1. **branch**, offshoot 2. support, sustain 3. protrude 4. pay	SI-7 (zhi zheng), TB-6 (zhi gou)
Zhì 至	1. arrive at, **reach** 2. until 3. extremely, **most**	B-67 (zhi yin), GV-9 (zhi yang)
Zhì 志	1. aspiration, ideal, **will** 2. mark, sign 3. annals, records 4. keep in mind	B-52 (zhi shi)

CHARACTER	MEANING	POINT NAME
Zhì 秩	arrangement, **order**, sequence	B-54 (*zhi bian*)
Zhōng 中	1. amidst, among 2. **center, middle** 3. China	L-1 (*zhong fu*), SI-15 (*jian zhong shu*), B-29 (*zhong lu shu*), B-40 (*wei zhong*), P-9 (*zhong chong*), TB-3 (*zhong zhu*), Liv-4 (*zhong feng*), Liv-6 (*zhong du*), CV-3 (*zhong ji*), CV-12 (*zhong wan*), CV-17 (*tan zhong*), GV-7 (*zhong shu*) GV-26 (*ren zhong*)
Zhōng 鐘	1. **bell** 2. clock 3. time 4. concentrate (one's affections) 5. (with the foot radical) the heel	K-4 (*da zhong*), G-39 (*xuan zhong*)
Zhú 竹	bamboo	B-2 (*zan zhu*), TB-23 (*si zhu kong*)
Zhǔ 渚	**islet**, sand bar	TB-3 (*zhong zhu*)
Zhù 杼	1. reed 2. (weaving) **shuttle**	B-11 (*da zhu*)
Zhù 柱	1. column, **pillar**, post 2. cylinder 3. support	B-10 (*tian zhu*), GV-12 (*shen zhu*)
Zhù 築	1. **sturdy** 2. (without the wood radical) a stringed muscial instrument 3. **build**, construct	K-9 (*zhu bin*)
Zhuī 椎	1. **vertebra** 2. hammer, mallet	GV-14 (*da zhui*), EX-9 (M-BW-25) (*shi qi zhui xia*)
Zǐ 子	1. tender, young 2. child, son 3. person 4. ancient title of respect for a learned or virtuous man 5. seed 6. **egg** 7. copper 8. first of the twelve earthly branches	G-1 (*tong zi liao*), EX-6 (M-CA-18) (*zi gong*)

CHARACTER	MEANING	POINT NAME
Zōng 宗	1. ancestor 2. **clan** 3. faction, religion, school, sect 4. principle, aim, purpose 5. model, master 6. follow, venerate, **worship**	SI-11 *(tian zong)*, TB-7 *(hui zong)*
Zú 足	foot	S-36 *(zu san li)*, B-66 *(zu tong gu)*, G-41 *(zu lin qi)*, G-44 *(zu qiao yin)*
Zuì 最	1. **extreme,** most 2. gather	L-6 *(kong zui)*

APPENDIX II

Point Index

**LUNG CHANNEL
OF HAND GREATER YIN**

L-1 (zhōng fǔ) Central Palace, 29
L-5 (chǐ zé) Cubit Marsh, 30
L-6 (kǒng zuì) Extreme Aperture, 31
L-7 (liè quē) Broken Sequence, 32
L-8 (jīng qú) Passing Ditch, 33
L-9 (tài yuān) Great Abyss, 34
L-10 (yú jì) Fish Border, 35
L-11 (shào shāng) Lesser Metal's Note, 36

**LARGE INTESTINE CHANNEL
OF HAND YANG BRIGHTNESS**

LI-1 (shāng yáng) Metal's Note Yang, 37
LI-2 (èr jiān) Second Interval, 38
LI-3 (sān jiān) Third Interval, 39
LI-4 (hé gǔ) Adjoining Valleys, 40
LI-5 (yáng xī) Yang Stream, 42
LI-6 (piān lì) Deviated Passage, 43
LI-7 (wēn liū) Temperate Flow, 44
LI-10 (shǒu sān lǐ) Arm Three Miles, 45
LI-11 (qū chí) Crooked Pool, 46
LI-14 (bì nào) Upper Arm's Musculature, 48
LI-15 (jiān yú) Shoulder's Corner, 49
LI-16 (jù gǔ) Giant Bone, 50
LI-18 (fú tū) Relieve Prominence, 51
LI-20 (yíng xiāng) Receiving Fragrance, 52

**STOMACH CHANNEL
OF FOOT YANG BRIGHTNESS**

S-1 (chéng qì) Contain Tears, 53
S-2 (sì bái) Four Brightness, 54
S-3 (jù liáo) Large Opening, 55
S-4 (dì cāng) Earth Granary, 56
S-6 (jiá chē) Jaw Vehicle, 57
S-7 (xià guān) Lower Hinge, 58
S-8 (tóu wéi) Skull's Safeguard, 59
S-9 (rén yíng) Man's Welcome, 60
S-18 (rǔ gēn) Breast Root, 61
S-21 (liáng mén) Connecting Gate, 62
S-25 (tiān shū) Heaven's Axis, 63
S-28 (shuǐ dào) Waterway, 65
S-29 (guī lái) Return, 66
S-30 (qì chōng) Qi's Breakthrough, 67
S-31 (bì guān) Hip's Border Gate, 68
S-32 (fú tù) Prostrate Rabbit, 69
S-34 (liáng qiū) Connecting Mound, 70
S-35 (dú bí) Calf's Nose, 71
S-36 (zú sān lǐ) Foot Three Miles, 72
S-37 (shàng jù xū) Upper Great Void, 75
S-38 (tiáo kǒu) Narrow Opening, 76
S-39 (xià jù xū) Lower Great Void, 77
S-40 (fēng lóng) Abundant Flourishing, 78
S-41 (jiě xī) Release Stream, 80
S-42 (chōng yáng) Rushing Yang, 81
S-43 (xiàn gǔ) Deep Valley, 82

Stomach Channel, CONT.

S-44 *(nèi tíng)* Inner Courtyard, 83
S-45 *(lì duì)* Evil's Dissipation, 84

SPLEEN CHANNEL OF FOOT GREATER YIN

Sp-1 *(yǐn bái)* Hidden Clarity, 85
Sp-2 *(dà dū)* Great Capital, 86
Sp-3 *(tài bái)* Great Brightness, 87
Sp-4 *(gōng sūn)* Ancestor and Descendant, 88
Sp-5 *(shāng qiū)* Metal's Note Hill, 90
Sp-6 *(sān yīn jiāo)* Three Yin Junction, 91
Sp-8 *(dì jī)* Earth's Mechanism, 93
Sp-9 *(yīn líng quán)* Yin Mound Spring, 94
Sp-10 *(xuè hǎi)* Sea of Blood, 95
Sp-12 *(chōng mén)* Penetrating Gate, 96
Sp-15 *(dà héng)* Great Transverse, 97
Sp-21 *(dà bāo)* Great Envelope, 98

HEART CHANNEL OF HAND LESSER YIN

H-1 *(jí quán)* Utmost Spring, 99
H-2 *(qīng líng)* Green Spirit, 100
H-3 *(shào hǎi)* Lesser Sea, 101
H-4 *(líng dào)* Spirit's Path, 102
H-5 *(tōng lǐ)* Communication's Route, 103
H-6 *(yīn xì)* Yin's Crevice, 104
H-7 *(shén mén)* Spirit's Gate, 105
H-8 *(shào fǔ)* Lesser Palace, 107
H-9 *(shào chōng)* Lesser Rushing, 108

SMALL INTESTINE CHANNEL OF HAND GREATER YANG

SI-1 *(shào zé)* Young Marsh, 109
SI-2 *(qián gǔ)* Forward Valley, 110
SI-3 *(hòu xī)* Back Stream, 111
SI-4 *(wàn gǔ)* Wrist Bone, 113
SI-5 *(yáng gǔ)* Yang Valley, 114
SI-6 *(yǎng lǎo)* Supporting the Old, 115
SI-7 *(zhī zhèng)* Branch from the Main, 116
SI-8 *(xiǎo hǎi)* Small Sea, 117
SI-9 *(jiān zhēn)* Shoulder Integrity, 118
SI-10 *(nào shū)* Scapula's Hollow, 119
SI-11 *(tiān zōng)* Heaven's Worship, 120
SI-12 *(bǐng fēng)* Holds Wind, 121
SI-15 *(jiān zhōng shū)* Middle Shoulder Hollow, 122
SI-17 *(tiān róng)* Heaven's Reception, 123
SI-18 *(quán liáo)* Cheekbone Opening, 124
SI-19 *(tīng gōng)* Palace of Hearing, 125

BLADDER CHANNEL OF FOOT GREATER YANG

B-1 *(jīng míng)* Eye's Clarity, 126
B-2 *(zǎn zhú)* Collection of Bamboo, 127
B-7 *(tōng tiān)* Penetrating Heaven, 128
B-10 *(tiān zhù)* Heaven's Pillar, 129
B-11 *(dà zhù)* Great Shuttle, 130
B-12 *(fēng mén)* Wind's Gate, 131
B-13 *(fèi shū)* Lung's Hollow, 132
B-14 *(jué yīn shū)* Absolute Yin Hollow, 133
B-15 *(xīn shū)* Heart's Hollow, 134
B-16 *(dū shū)* Governing Hollow, 135
B-17 *(gé shū)* Diaphragm's Hollow, 136
B-18 *(gān shū)* Liver's Hollow, 137
B-19 *(dǎn shū)* Gallbladder's Hollow, 139
B-20 *(pí shū)* Spleen's Hollow, 140
B-21 *(wèi shū)* Stomach's Hollow, 142
B-22 *(sān jiāo shū)* Triple Burner's Hollow, 143
B-23 *(shèn shū)* Kidney's Hollow, 144
B-24 *(qì hǎi shū)* Sea of Qi's Hollow, 146
B-25 *(dà cháng shū)* Large Intestine's Hollow, 147
B-26 *(guān yuán shū)* Hinge at the Source Hollow, 148
B-27 *(xiǎo cháng shū)* Small Intestine's Hollow, 149
B-28 *(páng guāng shū)* Bladder's Hollow, 150
B-29 *(zhōng lǔ shū)* Central Spine Hollow, 151
B-30 *(bái huán shū)* White Ring Hollow, 152
B-31~34 *(bā liáo)* Eight Foramina, 153
B-35 *(huì yáng)* Meeting of Yang, 154
B-36 *(chéng fú)* Bearing Support, 155
B-37 *(yīn mén)* Abundance Gate, 156
B-39 *(wěi yáng)* Entrusting Yang, 157
B-40 *(wěi zhōng)* Entrusting Middle, 158
B-42 *(pò hù)* Animal Soul Door, 160
B-43 *(gāo huāng shū)* Fatty Vital Hollow, 161
B-44 *(shén táng)* Spirit's Hall, 163
B-47 *(hún mén)* Spiritual Soul Gate, 164
B-49 *(yì shè)* Intelligence Lodge, 165

Bladder Channel, CONT.

B-52 (zhì shì) Will's Chamber, 166
B-54 (zhì biān) Order's Frontier, 167
B-57 (chéng shān) Supporting Mountain, 168
B-58 (fēi yáng) Flying Yang, 169
B-59 (fū yáng) Tarsal Yang, 170
B-60 (kūn lún) Kunlun Mountains, 171
B-61 (pú cān) Servant's Partaking, 172
B-62 (shēn mài) Extending Vessel, 173
B-63 (jīn mén) Golden Gate, 174
B-64 (jīng gǔ) Central Bone, 175
B-65 (shù gǔ) Restrained Bone, 176
B-66 (zú tōng gǔ) Foot Connecting Valley, 177
B-67 (zhì yīn) Reaching Yin, 178

KIDNEY CHANNEL
OF FOOT LESSER YIN

K-1 (yǒng quán) Gushing Spring, 179
K-2 (rán gǔ) Burning Valley, 180
K-3 (tài xī) Great Stream, 181-2
K-4 (dà zhōng) Large Bell, 183
K-5 (shuǐ quán) Water's Spring, 184
K-6 (zhào hǎi) Luminous Sea, 185
K-7 (fù liū) Repeated Current, 186
K-8 (jiāo xìn) Junction of Faithfulness, 187
K-9 (zhù bīn) Building for the Guest, 188
K-10 (yīn gǔ) Yin Valley, 189
K-27 (shū fǔ) Conveying Palace, 190

PERICARDIUM CHANNEL
OF HAND ABSOLUTE YIN

P-1 (tiān chí) Heaven's Pool, 191
P-2 (tiān quán) Heaven's Spring, 192
P-3 (qū zé) Curved Marsh, 193
P-4 (xì mén) Crevice Gate, 194
P-5 (jiān shǐ) Intermediary, 195
P-6 (nèi guān) Inner Border Gate, 196-7
P-7 (dà líng) Big Mound, 198
P-8 (láo gōng) Palace of Labor, 199
P-9 (zhōng chōng) Middle Rushing, 200

TRIPLE BURNER CHANNEL
OF HAND LESSER YANG

TB-1 (guān chōng) Gate's Rushing, 201
TB-2 (yè mén) Fluid's Door, 202
TB-3 (zhōng zhǔ) Middle Islet, 203
TB-4 (yáng chí) Yang's Pool, 204
TB-5 (wài guān) Outer Border Gate, 205
TB-6 (zhī gōu) Branch Ditch, 206
TB-7 (huì zōng) Assembly of the Clan, 207
TB-8 (sān yáng luò) Three Yang Connection, 208
TB-10 (tiān jǐng) Heaven's Well, 209
TB-14 (jiān liáo) Shoulder Opening, 210
TB-17 (yì fēng) Shielding Wind, 211
TB-21 (ěr mén) Ear's Gate, 212
TB-23 (sī zhú kōng) Silken Bamboo Hole, 213

GALLBLADDER CHANNEL
OF FOOT LESSER YANG

G-1 (tóng zǐ liáo) Pupil's Seam, 214
G-2 (tīng huì) Reunion of Hearing, 215
G-12 (wán gǔ) Completed Bone, 216
G-14 (yáng bái) Yang Brightness, 217
G-20 (fēng chí) Wind Pool, 218-9
G-21 (jiān jǐng) Shoulder Well, 220
G-24 (rì yuè) Sun and Moon, 221
G-25 (jīng mén) Capital Gate, 222
G-26 (dài mài) Girdle Vessel, 223
G-27 (wǔ shū) Five Pivots, 224
G-28 (wéi dào) Preserving Path, 225
G-29 (jū liáo) Inhabited Joint, 226
G-30 (huán tiào) Leaping Circumflexus, 227
G-31 (fēng shì) Wind's Market, 228
G-33 (xī yáng guān) Knee Yang Hinge, 229
G-34 (yáng líng quán) Yang Mound Spring, 230
G-35 (yáng jiāo) Yang's Intersection, 231
G-36 (wài qiū) Outer Mound, 232
G-37 (guāng míng) Bright Light, 233
G-38 (yáng fǔ) Yang's Assistant, 234
G-39 (xuán zhōng) Suspended Bell, 235
G-40 (qiū xū) Hill's Ruins, 236
G-41 (zú lín qì) Foot Verge of Tears, 237
G-43 (xiá xī) Brave Stream, 238
G-44 (zú qiào yīn) Foot Yin's Aperture, 239

LIVER CHANNEL
OF FOOT ABSOLUTE YIN

Liv-1 (dà dūn) Great Sincerity, 240
Liv-2 (xíng jiān) Travel Between, 241
Liv-3 (tài chōng) Great Thoroughfare, 242-3
Liv-4 (zhōng fēng) Middle Barrier, 244
Liv-5 (lí gōu) Draining Shells, 245
Liv-6 (zhōng dū) Central Capital, 246
Liv-8 (qū quán) Curved Spring, 247

Liver Channel, CONT.

Liv-13 (*zhāng mén*) Order Gate, 248
Liv-14 (*qī mén*) Gate of Hope, 249

CONCEPTION VESSEL

CV-1 (*huì yīn*) Meeting of Yin, 250
CV-2 (*qū gǔ*) Crooked Bone, 251
CV-3 (*zhōng jí*) Central Pole, 252
CV-4 (*guān yuán*) Hinge at the Source, 253-4
CV-5 (*shí mén*) Stone Gate, 255
CV-6 (*qì hǎi*) Sea of Qi, 256-7
CV-7 (*yīn jiāo*) Yin Junction, 258
CV-8 (*shén què*) Spirit's Palace Gate, 259
CV-9 (*shuǐ fēn*) Water Divide, 260
CV-10 (*xià wǎn*) Lower Stomach Cavity, 261
CV-11 (*jiàn lǐ*) Build Within, 262
CV-12 (*zhōng wǎn*) Middle Stomach Cavity, 263-4
CV-13 (*shàng wǎn*) Upper Stomach Cavity, 265
CV-14 (*jù què*) Great Palace Gate, 266
CV-15 (*jiū wěi*) Turtledove Tail, 267
CV-17 (*tán zhōng*) Central Altar, 268
CV-22 (*tiān tū*) Heaven's Chimney, 296
CV-23 (*lián quán*) Pure Spring, 270
CV-24 (*chéng jiāng*) Receiving Liquid, 271

GOVERNING VESSEL

GV-1 (*cháng qiáng*) Lasting Strength, 272
GV-2 (*yāo shū*) Lumbar's Hollow, 273
GV-3 (*yāo yáng guān*) Lumbar Yang's Hinge, 274
GV-4 (*mìng mén*) Vital Gate, 275-6
GV-5 (*xuán shū*) Suspended Axis, 277
GV-7 (*zhōng shū*) Central Axis, 278
GV-9 (*zhì yáng*) Supreme Yang, 279
GV-10 (*líng tái*) Spirit's Platform, 280
GV-11 (*shén dào*) Spirit Path, 281
GV-12 (*shēn zhù*) Body's Pillar, 282
GV-13 (*táo dào*) Moulded Path, 283
GV-14 (*dà zhuī*) Big Vertebra, 284
GV-15 (*yǎ mén*) Gate of Muteness, 285
GV-16 (*fēng fǔ*) Wind's Palace, 286
GV-17 (*nǎo hù*) Brain's Door, 287
GV-20 (*bǎi huì*) Hundred Meetings, 288-9
GV-23 (*shàng xīng*) Upper Star, 290
GV-26 (*rén zhōng*) Middle of Man, 291-2

EXTRAORDINARY POINTS

EX-1 (M-HN-3) (*yìn táng*) Seal Hall, 293
EX-2 (M-HN-9) (*tài yáng*) Sun, 294
EX-3 (M-HN-14) (*bí tōng*) Nose Passage, 295
EX-4 (M-HN-13) (*yì míng*) Shielding Brightness, 296
EX-5 (N-BW-21) (*ān mián*) Peaceful Sleep, 297
EX-6 (M-CA-18) (*zǐ gōng*) Womb, 298
EX-7 (M-BW-1) (*dìng chuǎn*) Stop Wheezing, 299
EX-8 (M-BW-24) (*yāo yǎn*) Lumbar's Aperture, 300
EX-9 (M-BW-25) (*shí qī zhuī xià*) Below 17 Vertebrae, 301
EX-10 (M-BW-35) (*huá tuó jiā jǐ*) Hua Tuo Bilateral Spinal Points, 302
EX-11 (M-UE-9) (*sì fèng*) Four Seams, 303
EX-12 (M-UE-22) (*bā xié*) Eight Evils, 304
EX-13 (M-UE-1) (*shí xuān*) Ten Drainings, 305
EX-14 (M-UE-48) (*jiān nèi líng*) Shoulder's Inner Tomb, 306
EX-15 (M-LE-8) (*bā fēng*) Eight Winds, 307
EX-16 (M-LE-13) (*lán wěi*) Appendix, 308
EX-17 (M-LE-23) (*dǎn náng*) Gallbladder, 309

BIBLIOGRAPHY

Banever, Robert. *The Points of Chinese Acupuncture*. Published by the author, 1977.

Beijing College of Chinese Medicine. *English Dictionary of Chinese Medical Terms*. Beijing: The People's Medical Publishing House, 1979.

Beijing College of Traditional Chinese Medicine, comp. *Essentials of Chinese Acupuncture*. Beijing: Foreign Languages Press, 1980.

Birch, Stephen, and Kiiko Matsumoto. *Extraordinary Vessels*. Brookline: Paradigm Publications, 1986.

Birch, Stephen, and Kiiko Matsumoto. *Five Elements and Ten Stems*. Higganum: Paradigm Publications, 1986.

Blofield, John. *Taoism: The Quest for Immortality*. London: Unwin Paperbacks, 1979.

Chan, Po-tuan. *The Inner Teachings of Taoism*. Translated by Thomas Cleary. Boston: Shambhala Publications, 1986.

Chen Jing. *Anatomical Atlas of Chinese Acupuncture Points*. Jinan: Shandong Science and Technology Press, 1982.

Chia, Mantak. *Awaken Healing Energy Through the Tao: The Taoist Secret of Circulating Internal Power*. New York: Aurora Press, 1983.

Cleary, Thomas. *The Taoist I Ching*. Boston: Shambhala Publications, 1986.

Cooper, J. C. *Chinese Alchemy: The Taoist Quest for Immortality*. Wellingborough: The Aquarian Press, 1984.

Coward, Harold. *Jung and Eastern Thought*. Albany: State University of New York Press, 1985.

Darras, Jean-Claude. *Transliterations of the Chinese Acupuncture Point Names with Explanations. Vol. 1 (Traite d'Acuponcture Medicale, Tome 1)*. Translated by Michael C. Barnett. Miami: Occidental Institute of Chinese Studies, 1983.

Deadman, Peter. "The Actions of the Acupuncture Points". The Journal of Chinese Medicine 18-21 (1985-6).

DeWoskin, Kenneth J. *Doctors, Diviners, and Magicians of Ancient China: Biographies of Fang-Shih*. New York: Columbia University Press, 1983.

East Asian Medical Studies Society. *Fundamentals of Chinese Medicine*. Brookline: Paradigm Publications, 1985.

Flaws, Bob. *The Path of Pregnancy*. Brookline: Paradigm Publications, 1983.

Hoare, Sophy. *Yoga*. London: MacDonald Educational, 1977.

Huang, Xiaokia, and Zhufan Xie, ed. *Dictionary of Traditional Chinese Medicine*. Hong Kong: Commercial Press, 1984.

Huard, Pierre, and Ming Wong. *Chinese Medicine*. Translated by Bernard Fielding. New York: McGraw-Hill, 1968.

Ki, Sunu, and Yunkyo Lee. *Huang di nei jing ling shu: The Canon of Acupuncture*. Seoul: Hong Sung Enterprises, 1985.

Kinoshita, Haruto. *Illustration of Acupoints*. Tokyo: Ido no nippon sha, 1970.

Larre, Claude, Jean Schatz, and Elizabeth Rochat De La Vallee. *Survey of Traditional Chinese Medicine*. Translated by S.E. Stang. Paris and Columbia: Institut Ricci and the Traditional Acupuncture Foundation, 1986.

Lawson-Wood, D., and J. Lawson-Wood. *Acupuncture Vitality & Revival Points*. Devon: Health Science Press, 1960.

Leung, K. Y. "Chinese Medical Philosophy and Principles of Diagnosis". Salem: North American College of Acupuncture. Course notes 1, 1971.

Leung, K. Y. "Acupuncture Points and Techniques". Salem: North American College of Acupuncture. Course notes 2, 1971.

Low, Royston. *The Celestial Stems: Acupuncture Theory and Practice in Relation to the Influence of Cosmic Forces Upon the Body*. New York: Thorsons Publishers, 1985.

Lu K'uan Yu. *The Secrets of Chinese Meditation*. New York: Samuel Weiser, 1964.

Manaka, Yoshio, and Ian A. Urquhart. *The Layman's Guide to Acupuncture*. New York: John Weatherhill, 1972.

Motoyama, Hiroshi. *Theories of the Chakra: Bridge to Higher Consciousness*. Wheaton: Theosophical Publishing House, 1981.

Needham, J. *Science and Civilization in China*. Vol. 3, *Mathematics and the Sciences of the Heavens and the Earth*. Cambridge: Cambridge University Press, 1959.

Nguyen, D. Hiep. *The Dictionary of Acupuncture and Moxibustion*. Rochester: Thorsons Publishing, 1987.

Omura, Yoshiaki. *Acupuncture Medicine: It's Historical and Clinical Background*. Tokyo: Japan Publications, 1982.

Player, Graham. *Disease and Diagnosis for the Acupuncturist: An Advanced Guide to Traditional Diagnostic Techniques*. New York: Thorsons Publishers, 1984.

Ross, Jeremy. *Zang Fu: The Organ Systems of Traditional Chinese Medicine*. Edinburgh: Churchill Livingstone, 1984.

Shanghai College of Traditional Medicine. *Acupuncture: A Comprehensive Text*. Translated and edited by John O'Connor and Dan Bensky. Chicago: Eastland Press, 1981.

So, James Tin Yau. *The Book of Acupuncture Points: Volume One of A Complete Course in Acupuncture*. Brookline: Paradigm Publications, 1985.

Unschuld, Paul U., trans. and annot. *Nan-Ching: The Classic of Difficult Issues*. Berkeley: University of California Press, 1986.

Unschuld, Paul U. *Medicine in China: A History of Ideas*. Berkeley: University of California Press, 1985.

Veith, Ilza, trans. *Huang Ti Nei Ching Su Wen: The Yellow Emperor's Classic of Internal Medicine*. Berkeley: University of California Press, 1949.

Welch, H., and A. Seidel. *Facets of Taoism: Essays in Chinese Religion*. New Haven: Yale University Press, 1979.

Wieger, L., and L. Davrout, trans. *Chinese Characters: Their Origin, Etymology, History, Classification and Signification*. New York: Paragon Book Reprint Corp. and Dover Publications, 1965.

Wilder, G. D., and J. H. Ingram. *Analysis of Chinese Characters*. New York: Dover Publications, 1922.

Wilhelm, Hellmut. *Change: Eight Lectures on the I Ching*. Translated by Cary F. Baynes. Princeton: Princeton University Press, 1960.

Wilhelm, Hellmut. *Heaven, Earth, and Man in the Book of Changes*. Seattle: University of Washington Press, 1977.

Wilhelm, Richard. *The I Ching or Book of Changes*. Translated by Cary F. Baynes. New York: Bollingen Foundation, 1950.

Wu, Jingrong, ed. *The Pinyin Chinese-English Dictionary*. New York and Hong Kong: John Wiley & Sons and Commercial Press, 1979.

Xia, Chong-xin. "Functions of the Major Acupuncture Points". Beijing: Department of Acupuncture, Guan An Men Hospital, n.d.

Li, Xuewu, and Meng Ziankun, trans., Yang, Jiasan, ed. *The Way to Locate Acu-points*. Beijing: Foreign Languages Press, 1982.

Zhang, Rui-fu, Xiu-fen Wu, and Nissi S. Wang. *Illustrated Dictionary of Chinese Acupuncture*. Hong Kong and Beijing: Sheep's Publications and People's Medical Publishing House, 1985.

Zhou, Mei-sheng. *Translation of Names of the Acupoints – with English Translation*. Translated by Shi-tai Huang and Zai-yi Zhang. Hefei: Anhui Publishing House of Science and Technology, 1985.

Chinese Texts:

Gao, Shi-guo. *Interpretations of the Acupuncture Point Names (Zhen jiu xue ming jie)*. Harbin: Heilongjiang Science and Technology Press, 1985.

Gao, Wu. *Gatherings from Outstanding Acupuncturists (Zhen jiu ju ying)*. Shanghai: Shanghai Science and Technology Press,1961.

Huang-Fu, Mi. *Systematic Classic of Acupuncture and Moxibustion (Zhen jiu jia yi jing)*. Commercial Affairs Press, 1955.

Li, Shi-zhen. *Clinical Developments on the Commonly Used Acupuncture Points (Chang yong shu xue lin chuang fa hui)*. Beijing: People's Health Publishing Co., 1985.

Ma, Shi. *Correct Meaning of the Classic of Difficulties (Nan jing zhen yi)*. Shanghai: Shanghai Science and Technology Press, 1981.

Qi, Gan. *A Compilation of Acupuncture Point Name Interpretations (Jing xue shi yi hui jie)*. Shanghai: Shanghai Translation Publishing Co, 1984.

Sun, Si-miao. *Supplement of the Thousand Ducat Prescriptions (Qian jin yao fang)*. Beijing: People's Health Publishing Co., 1955.

Wang, Wei-yi. *llustrated Classic of Acupuncture Points on the Bronze Model (Tong ren zhen jiu shu xue tu jing)*. Beijing: People's Health Publishing Co., 1955.

Wang, Zhi-zheng. *Classic of Nourishing Life with Acupuncture and Moxibustion (Zhen jiu zi sheng jing)*. Shanghai: Shanghai Science and Technology Press, 1959.

Yang, Ji-zhou. *Great Compendium of Acupuncture and Moxibustion (Zhen jiu da cheng)*. Beijing: People's Health Publishing Co., 1963.

Yellow Emperor's Inner Classic (Huang di nei jing). Beijing: People's Health Publishing Co., 1964.